HOLISTIC
HOME

The Homemaker's Guide
to Health and Happiness

HOLISTIC HOME

The Homemaker's Guide
to Health and Happiness

Maxine Fox

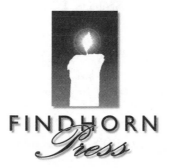

FINDHORN
Press

First published in English by Findhorn Press 2006

ISBN 10: 1-84409-070-1
ISBN 13: 978-1-84409-070-9

British Library Cataloguing-in-Publication Data.
A catalogue record for this book is available
from the British Library.

Edited by Kate Keogan
Cover and interior design by Damian Keenan

Printed and bound by WS Bookwell, Finland

Published by
Findhorn Press
305a The Park, Findhorn
Forres IV36 3TE
Scotland, UK

Telephone
01309 - 690582
Fax
01309 - 690036

info@findhornpress.com
www.findhornpress.com

For my Dad
Kindness as Inspiration

Contents

1. Introduction   1
   How the home evolved... the need for respite... alchemy
2. Before We Begin   5
   Consumerism... the issue of waste... ways to reduce, re-use and recycle

SECTION 1

3. Building Firm Foundations   12
   Sick building syndrome... indoor pollutants... what you can do
4. Cleaning Up Your Home the Chemical-free Way   16
   Non toxic approaches to healthy house-keeping
5. Beauty and the Beast   21
   The natural path to health and beauty
6. What We Eat   27
   *The problems with intensive farming... the case for organic...
   a return to common sense*
7. How We Eat   32
   Rituals and sharing... spiritual sustenance
8. How We Recognize and Resolve Physical Discomfort   35
   Ergonomic assessment... practical applications
9. Ease and Dis-ease   39
   The mind/body connection... the power of belief... initiating healing

SECTION 2

10. Creating Health   44
    The happiness factor... self-responsibility... health and harmony
11. Making Sense of Design   48
    *Intuitive responses... Sacred Geometry... design and placement...
    clutter confronted*
12. Colour Conscious   54
    *Colour energy... nutrition for mind and body...chakras...
    colour messages*
13. Light As Therapy   65
    The healing power of the Sun... lighting solutions for your home
14. The Sensual Home   70
    Creating harmony through texture, aroma and sound

15. Essential Elements   79
    Earth, fire, water and air: colours, imagery and materials
16. Inspiration   87
    Creativity…catharsis…clarity
17. Connection   91
    Universal truths…balance…sustainability…respect

SECTION 3

18. Active Healing   98
    Consciousness… our pack mentality… the need for inclusion
19. Family and Friends   104
    Investment and reward… the importance of play…
    negotiation… self-respect
20. From Home to Community   107
    Neighbours… community spirit… team building
21. The Market-Place   111
    Responsibility… resonance… fair trade… ethical consumerism
22. Our Global Home   120
    The environment… natural resources… the need for redress
23. Animal Magic   130
    Animal welfare… the legacy we are creating…
    the lessons we could learn
24. The Natural Garden   138
    Nature's wonderland… companion planting…
    herbs, health and diversity
25. The Turning of the Year   144
    Celtic traditions… seasons, festivals and celebrations…
    re-birth and renewal
26. The Cosmos   153
    The cosmic triumvirate… the importance of three…
    paradigms and possibilities
27. The Self / The Whole   156
    Science and intuition… the power of intention…
    the future in our hands.

    Appendices   163
    References, bibliography, useful addresses.

PLEASE NOTE

The advice given in this book is for general guidance only and is not intended to take the place of individualized treatment by a qualified health practitioner. Any application of the ideas offered herein is at the reader's sole risk and discretion.

CHAPTER 1

❀ ❀ ❀   # Introduction   ❀ ❀ ❀

During the thousands of years of our evolution, our homes have served a simple but fundamental need: that of protection. Since our earliest beginnings, the world that has fed and clothed us has also been full of hostile forces: animals and outsider groups that might attack and weather that could freeze, scorch, soak or smother. As they sought reprieve from these elements, our primitive ancestors took refuge in caves and temporary shelters which in time they began to adorn with flowers, shells, stones and later, to decorate with primitive art. The caves at Lascaux, in South West France, are richly furnished with paintings of horses, buffalo and deer that date back as far as 18,000BC but why exactly did pre-historic men and women feel the need to invest such time and energy in this seemingly non-essential activity? What motivated early humans to transform the den from mere practical shelter into a home?

The answer lies within our basic physiology. Our stress response, that is to say the flight or fight response is a well-honed survival device that forms part of our own and indeed all animals' physiology. As a short-term measure, these responses serve to heighten our physical abilities, allowing us to escape from or avoid threatening situations. However, the body is unable to maintain this stress response for any sustained period of time without impinging on its ability to remain healthy. It is only by ensuring periods of relaxation that balance can be restored and good health maintained in the long term. This tells us that our need for respite is as much a part of our evolutionary success as is our ability to deal with stress. It remains as true today as it has always been that, in order to thrive, it is imperative that we take the time to relax.

Originally, our predecessors were free to locate this personal refuge wherever they felt was appropriate, choosing somewhere that spoke to them of its inherent natural qualities: secure, sheltered, of sympathetic size and auspicious location. But as these hunter-gatherer ancestors evolved into a society of farmers, land inevitably became linked to wealth and prestige. Our primeval fear of being left behind was distilled into a desire to curry favour with those in power; land and the wealth that it bequeathed became the currency of choice. This led society to regard property as proof of success and it is still the case today that, for most people, the biggest material investment is the home.

The primal hunger which once drove us to hunt for food and shelter has since mutated into a full-volume quest for the perfect lifestyle, resulting in an explosion of interest in home renovation, refurbishment, D.I.Y and quick-fix remedies. The relentless pressure to upgrade has been reinforced by the endless property development programmes that dominate prime time television; the racks of magazines and books devoted to everything from architecture to needlepoint; the emergence of every kind of design professional and supply superstore all of which offer endless choices, trends, 'must haves' and opportunities for mistakes, disasters and financial ruin. Unfortunately, the more we focus on aesthetic trends and notions of status, the less likely we are to create a home that meets our true need, which is to ensure our health and happiness. The subtle yet profound impact that the home environment has on our physical and emotional being tends to be overlooked by many, including conventional architects and designers. But, in truth, it is in the realm of interaction (rather than simple aesthetics) that the alchemy of turning a house into a home really happens.

The fact of this interaction becomes apparent to us through the intuitive responses we have to any given environment. Some rooms feel immediately comfortable and we are happy to linger, while others seem to be designed with the sole intention of moving us on. As far as one's own home is concerned, the nature of this interaction is shaped by the multitude of choices made (both consciously and subconsciously) regarding all aspects of homemaking. This two-way effect means that our homes reveal far more about us than we realize, being both a reflection and an expression of our innermost state of being. As our spiritual and emotional being dwells within our physical body, so we dwell within our home: in comfort or otherwise. Therefore the aim of this book is not to offer yet more guidance on aesthetic trends or tricks of the design trade, but rather to re-focus our attention on the interaction that occurs between our physical, emotional and spiritual selves and the living environment we call home.

The pre-occupation with materialism that dominates our society's attitude towards success is mirrored in its attitude towards physical health. The Western approach to healthcare tends to focus on the material manifestations of disease and dysfunction, i.e. its signs and symptoms, while encouraging us to ignore the subtle mental and emotional imbalances that should alert us to impending crisis. However, prevention is always preferable to cure so the first step in establishing a holistically healthy home is to create one that does us no physical damage in the first place. It may seem strange that the very place we think of as a sanctuary could be implicated in causing physical ill-health and impairment, but the toxic nature of many of the products within the home is such that this is very often the case. Add to this the discomfort caused by poorly-designed or sagging furniture, as well as ill-fitted or inadequately maintained appliances and, all in all, our homes have the potential to do more harm than good. Maximizing the degree of physical support given by the home lays the foundation upon which holistic health can then be built.

The sad fact is that, despite our society enjoying a higher standard of living than at any previous time in our history, rather than being well off, as a nation we are chronically unwell. Improvements to housing and sanitation, in conjunction with the discovery of antibiotics, may have afforded a temporary victory over some of the killers of yesteryear, but in the meantime we have managed to generate a whole catalogue of diseases that were simply not prevalent a few generations ago. Heart disease, cancer, asthma, diabetes, obesity and depression are all indicators of a society and a people under severe emotional and environmental stress. But it is only as our understanding of the human immune response mechanism evolves that the importance of emotional wellbeing in maintaining good physical health is starting to be recognized. Once again, the home has a crucial role to play; as the pressures of 21st century survival increase, it is the home that can offer the perfect antidote. By becoming aware of the very real physical and psychological effects initiated by design, colour and lighting, we can begin to make choices within the home that actively support our good health. Having done so, our homes become more than just a place to hang our hat: they acquire the active power to heal.

By consciously making the home a more healing environment, we reassert one of its most fundamental roles, which is to nurture the family bond. Today, the home may take many forms and play host to many types of family but the need to strengthen this clan connection remains primary. As external pressures increase, forcing many to spend more and more time outside the family circle, the role of the home as a facilitator of relationships is often forgotten. But it is only by honouring the fundamental importance of the den and the sense of kinship it encapsulates that we can hope to ensure the wellbeing of the individual, the family and of society as a whole. For this reason, the holistic home will always give high priority to the emotional needs of the family it embraces; in this way we find the happiness which is the key to accessing true wellbeing.

Having secured personal happiness, one is better able look beyond one's own needs to the needs of others: finally able to travel beyond the primal drive for survival, or the ego-instigated desire to acquire wealth and prestige, to arrive at a place of faith. When acting 'in good faith', choices are made whose benefits may never become apparent to the individual; they are nevertheless decided upon in the belief that, ultimately, they will act for the highest good of all. Within the home, this means bringing conscious awareness to the true (but often hidden) costs inherent in much of the produce and merchandise that goes to make up our lifestyle. Only when we, as individuals, stop giving priority to the needs of the self and begin instead to act with the uppermost regard for all life will we be able to open the door to the unseen but ultimate source of holistic good health.

Such is the potential for health and happiness inherent within the home that we can harness it to effect the process of positive change: towards health, towards happiness, towards humanity. This change can come about without financial outlay, without downsizing (unless we wish to), without major upheaval; it just involves taking a fresh look at what we have, what our options are and what we truly need from life.

What follows, then, is a way of re-creating our homes in such a way as to allow healing to manifest on all levels: the physical, the emotional and the spiritual. Homes that work to support our physical health rather than causing us harm as many do at present. Homes that encourage awareness and harmony within our relationships. Homes that allow us to re-connect to our selves, to each other, to nature: the truly holistic home.

CHAPTER 2

Before We Begin

Before we can begin to draw together the many threads that constitute the holistic home, it is first necessary to acknowledge the impact that any refurbishment or renewal is going to have on the environment. All new and replacement items will impact on our environment in some way so, before doing anything, we need to take a moment to assess what really needs to be done. Is there anything that can be modified, repaired, renovated or cleaned up, rather than simply discarded and replaced anew? Of course, these actions will also carry their environmental costs but, by striving to use only ecologically-friendly products, the amount of new toxins that leach into our world can be minimized.

Although the notion of recycling unwanted items is beginning to catch on, it is the mania for buying new products that is the primary cause for concern. Now that consumerism has replaced window-shopping as a national pastime, all that is deemed no longer state of the art, the height of convenience or is in less than perfect condition is being thrown out with the trash. As a consequence, we find ourselves drowning in a sea of rubbish, with pressure on landfill sites at an all time high, ever more incinerators proposed and an infestation of rats that thrive on our filthy habits. It is high time that we, as a society, got to grips with the issue of rubbish.

Manufacturers are partly responsible, having instigated a wily marketing strategy which, since the 1950s, has aimed to limit the life-span of everything from toasters to washing machines. Furthermore, as the speed of technological development advances, proud new owners frequently find that they have just got their new gadget home only to discover that an improved model has since been unveiled. The combination of these two factors has sowed the seeds of the retail mania that has since come to overwhelm us.

The problem of what to do with unwanted electrical items (such as televisions, computers, microwaves and music systems) has now become such a cause for concern that governments around the world are finally taking steps to force manufacturers to become more responsible for the toxic waste which they ultimately create.

It is only by ignoring the long-term environmental costs inherent in the production (and eventual dismantling) of such items that manufacturers have made these once-luxury goods not only affordable but commonplace, with some homes owning two, three or even more audio-visual units. The need to address this issue is especially pressing where computers are concerned as, not only are they increasingly common in both the home and the workplace, but they have the highest turnover rate of any electrical equipment. This represents a vast and highly toxic waste problem, involving billions of pounds of lead, cadmium, hexavalent chromium and mercury. Similar hazardous chemicals are found in mobile phones, with the seepage from a single unit capable of polluting 600,000 litres of water.

Behind the eye-catching slogans offering bargains and cut-price deals lies a hidden cost, one that is being left for the environment and the future to pick up. The production, manufacturing and disposal of textiles, for example, carries a particularly high price-tag. Chemical dyes use substances such as naphthalene, a known carcinogen, as well as bleaching agents and mordants, all of which add to pollution levels by leaching into the air, soil and ground water. Added to this is the environmental impact of transportation (often across several continents in the name of cheaper production costs) and, finally, the landfill problems that occur once these items are discarded. It is possible to recycle textiles through second-hand and charity shops, but this does not eliminate the ultimate problem of what to do with waste fabric, furnishing and carpets. Although natural fibres such as coir, cotton or wool will eventually biodegrade, little data exists on the time and implications involved. What is known is that the methane emitted during breakdown significantly adds to levels already present in the atmosphere. Synthetic fibres have to be chemically recycled in order to extract what is useful, so this option also has environmental repercussions.

Within the home, we have been encouraged by manufacturers to leave behind quaint pastimes like mending and restoration and to embrace instead the concept of the trend, an idea more traditionally associated with the fashion industry. The carpentry and joinery skills that once created furniture to last for generations have been replaced with mass-produced, chipboard assemblages that are ready for the scrapheap within just a few years. Curtains faded by the Sun are more likely to be replaced than re-dyed, while sofas and armchairs that would once have been re-upholstered are now discarded and replaced. All of this perfectly suits manufacturers who are more interested in the profits ensured by the replacement market than in fostering a reputation based on quality production.

Society needs to radically reassess this throwaway culture because, whether we choose to acknowledge it or not, it constitutes a very serious threat to our green and pleasant land. Whilst governments are starting to respond with waste strategies aimed at increasing rates of household and commercial recycling, it is ultimately down to us as individuals to change our lazy ways and take steps towards a less waste-congested future.

The most useful step to take is simply to opt out of the whole consumer madness of endlessly buying stuff in the first place. It is an indictment of our times that, having spent vast sums in accumulating our possessions, some are then prepared to spend even more money to have someone come in and de-clutter their homes. When you do need to buy something, do some research in order to ascertain which product has the best environmental credentials. For household appliances, check in terms of energy efficiency, reliability, performance, use of easily recyclable materials, potential for up-grading without replacing, even the amount of packaging used and choose the best quality product that you can afford. For consumers, these criteria offer by far the best long-term value for money, both for our pockets and our environmental future. Consumer magazines, environmental watchdogs, government-backed energy efficiency advice centres and even the companies themselves now offer information on which products are environmentally friendly. Another option is to log on to the internet and see what it has to offer. Many ecologically-aware companies only advertise and sell through this medium, meaning that the choice available is actually far greater than may be apparent when walking around the shops. Manufacturers are primarily concerned with endorsement by the paying public so by choosing only those products with sound environmental and ethical credentials, we can begin to effect a direct influence on the policy-making of the manufacturing world.

When it comes to buying furniture, the properties of real wood are hard to beat but do ensure that any new wooden furniture carries the Forest Stewardship Council label, guaranteeing that it comes from carefully managed sources. Better still, make use of the vast reserve of used furniture available from second-hand shops, reclamation yards and antique markets. Here you will be able to find fairly-priced pieces which are frequently of a better quality material and craftsmanship than can be found in the mass-market sector.

On a day-to-day basis, become aware of yet another marketing ploy: the 'convenience' con, those use-once-and-discard products designed to offer us short-term gains in time but with long-term repercussions that include environmental destruction, toxic waste and health impairment.

A major culprit is the disposable nappy. The Women's Environmental Network has estimated that British households throw away nearly 8 million disposable nappies every single day, with 90% of them going straight into landfill sites. Although exact figures are unknown, the plastic found in each one of these chemical-filled time capsules could take hundreds of years to decompose. Despite persuasive marketing campaigns, the only advantage that disposables (for which one should read 'hide-ables') have over real nappies is convenience for the parent. Contrary to the widespread belief that disposable nappies help prevent nappy rash, there is in fact little difference, in terms of prevention, between these and washable nappies. The big difference is that, whereas washable nappies can be used again and again, today's thoughtlessly discarded disposable could still be clogging up ever more valued land space when your new-born's great, great grandchildren are starting school.

Alternatively the re-usable nappy comes with biodegradable one-way liners that can be removed and the contents flushed away, leaving the cloth itself to be washed at 60 degrees for total hygiene: good for baby, good for their future. Remember that, however hard the marketing strategists may try to tempt us, the truth is that there is absolutely nothing convenient or life-enhancing about the environmental pollution caused by the array of disposable items that we are told we cannot live without.

With any product, we need to consider not just the item we buy but its packaging as well. Every year billions and billions of plastic bottles, bags, tubs and wrappers find their way to landfill sites around the world, their disposable nature blinding us to the true cost to the environment. Aluminium cans and glass bottles are relatively easy to recycle as many communities now have access to communal bins if not actual doorstep collection, but they are expensive in terms of production and transportation. Paper or card bags and cartons can be transported flat to the food manufacturer, thus reducing transportation costs and, as they are made primarily of wood from managed forests, they provide a renewable, recyclable and environmentally low-impact option. Supermarkets are starting to take this issue seriously and some are even investing in biodegradable, compostable packaging, so try to support this practice where you see it. As a further measure, buy in bulk where appropriate or check to see if a refill facility is available. Finally, ensure that you begin any shopping trip armed with enough carrier bags to meet your purchasing requirements. Plastic bags only came into being 25 years ago but thanks to their ubiquity have become such a recognized nuisance that countries from Australia to Ireland have begun taxing or even banning them outright. In Ireland, the new tax caused a reduction in their usage by 95%, showing what can be done with the right incentive. The Bag for Life scheme, begun by the UK supermarket chain Waitrose in 1997, has become widely adopted in other food halls but remember to take bags for other retail trips, too.

Try to incorporate some kind of recycling and sorting area, either within the kitchen itself or just outside the back door. A set of pull-out drawers (such as those designed for children's rooms) are useful for this, being hard-wearing, easy to keep clean and neat to transport to the recycling station. Paper, foil, tin cans, glass and plastic bottles, cardboard, plastic bags as well as textiles, books and shoes can all be recycled, while vegetable and garden waste can go on the compost heap to provide nutrients for your plants the following year. For more specialist waste such as paint, mobile phones, computers and white appliances contact the local council or get in touch with one of the many national and international recycling schemes that take our unwanted items and re-issue them for the benefit of others.

Although the environmental benefits of resisting the urge to buy in the first place and then recycling are decidedly long-term, by doing so you will be making a serious gesture towards a cleaner future. By affirming your commitment to the environment, you will send a wake-up call to manufacturers concerning the expectations we have of them and of our future. This self-empowered reclamation of our planet is of fundamental importance if we are to reach our goal of continuing good health; with these thoughts in mind, let's begin our re-assessment of our lifestyles and take the first step towards creating a more holistically supportive home.

Section 1

THE PHYSICAL
HOME

CHAPTER 3

Building Firm Foundations

Any house is only as strong as the foundations upon which it is built; where the holistic home is concerned, those foundations are created with the primary objective of supporting our physical health. Only by ensuring the health of our own most basic building block, i.e. the cells of our physical bodies, can a truly healthy home then manifest.

The first step is to ensure that the house is not causing any actual physical harm. Such are the levels of toxicity carried by many of the products and materials found in the average home that they are causing very real problems for our health. According to the US Environmental Protection Agency (EPA), indoor air pollutants have been ranked amongst the top five environmental risks to public health. Studies by the EPA have shown that levels of pollutants indoors can be two to five times greater than those outdoors, rising on occasion to as much as 100 times greater[1]. The problems caused by these pollutants are exacerbated by the fact that we are all spending more and more time indoors. Children are at particular risk because they breathe a greater volume of air in relation to their body size than do adults. Reducing the amount of toxins that our bodies are expected to deal with is therefore the number one priority and the first area to look at with regard to this is the infrastructure of the home itself.

The paint, plaster, varnishes, carpets, textiles and appliances that adorn your home can inadvertently be the cause of serious health problems including irritation of the nose, throat and lungs; increased risk of respiratory infections; nausea; tiredness; back, neck and eye strain; even fits. More subtle, but just as debilitating, are the psychological effects of depression, irritability, poor concentration and lethargy. These symptoms have been collectively recognized as sick building syndrome. The suspected reason for their emergence is that, as a response to increased pressure on fuel resources, since the 1970s architects have been encouraged to create sealed spaces for us to live and work in. These allow for a reduction in heating costs but encourage an increase in the build up of airborne toxins. Noxious fumes (including benzene from paint and formaldehyde from furnishing and insulation materials) then become increasingly concentrated through the use of air conditioning systems.

Industry soon cottoned on to sick building syndrome, as studies show that it continues to contribute to a significant reduction in productivity as well as a substantial rise in absenteeism. These effects can be just as damaging in the domestic arena as here, too, people have been encouraged to double glaze and insulate their homes against noise, the weather and potential intruders.

Floors and walls are sealed against wear and tear and the elements while changing fashions mean that open chimneys, which once allowed for a continuous change of air throughout day and night, are frequently boarded up.

Although the need for ventilation is generally pandered to when applying new paints and varnishes, remember that most new fabrics, furnishings, floor coverings and insulation materials also give off toxic particles that need to be cleared. The advice is that if you are planning to move into a newly-built, newly-decorated home, you should open all the windows and switch the heating on full in order to hasten the evaporation of any toxins before the family arrives. Of course, this has its own environmental impact so before making any decisions, it is worth becoming aware of the literal headaches caused by the home environment and of some of the more ecologically friendly alternatives available.

Paint contains what are known as volatile organic compounds (VOCs). These toxic elements evaporate quickly, thus allowing the paint to dry. Oil-based paints tend to have a higher VOC content than water-based paints and, for this reason, should be avoided. It is possible to buy absorbers (made from aluminium silicate) to which the VOC compounds stick; better yet, choose from one of the wide range of non-toxic paints now available from specialist manufacturers. If the ready-mixed, non-toxic paints are too expensive for you, a compromise can be achieved by using a non-toxic match-pot diluted with water to make a colour wash for use over a cheaper, non-toxic white or cream background. Alternatively, use a paddle attachment on an electric drill to mix a large pot of non-toxic white with a non-toxic match-pot of a tone several shades deeper than the colour you want to achieve.

By using water-based paints and glazes, the walls themselves are allowed to breathe. In turn, this through passage of air and moisture helps to regulate the atmosphere inside the home. A word of warning though: many people don't bother to wear rubber gloves when using water-based products as they are easily washed off with soap and water. However, these products are much more readily absorbed into the skin than are oil-based ones and so must be used with similar caution.

Formaldehyde is another chemical common in products destined for the home: it is found in commercial fibreboard (MDF), in plaster, in floor covering, in furniture adhesives as well as in foam insulation material, manmade fibres and dyes. Used as a biological preservative, over-exposure to this substance can lead to eye, ear, nose and lung irritation and possibly even to cancer. Fortunately, there are alternatives. Low formaldehyde-emission particleboard is readily available but the best option is to use non-toxic fibreboards made from waste wheat straw or woody material and fixed with natural wood resin. These are lighter in weight and generally more resistant to moisture penetration. Lime, clay and natural gypsum make a less toxic alternative to ordinary plaster and plasterboard. However, if these are not an option, ensure that your regular plaster or fibreboard is primed with a specialist non-toxic binding solution in order to prevent emissions from irritating the eyes, nose and throat.

Although a wide variety of natural fibres are now available for floor coverings, many still contain a veritable cocktail of harmful chemicals including pesticides, fungicides and synthetic dyes. Added to this heady mix are stain-inhibiting treatments, synthetic latex underlay and chemical adhesives; if you or any of your family are sensitive to synthetic chemicals, be sure to check the small print beyond the '100% natural' label. Truly environmentally friendly flooring (including seagrass, sisal and wool) is available from specialist companies and can be used for carpeting in conjunction with cotton, jute or hessian underlay. For those with allergies to lanolin or dust mites, linoleum, wood, cork or bamboo will make for a surface that is hard-wearing but supportive underfoot. Fabrics like linen, hessian, wool and cotton can be used for soft furnishings (including furniture coverings and curtaining), while more delicate natural fibres, such as muslin and lace, can be used for throws and cushions. Although some of these alternatives may seem expensive in comparison to the synthetics on offer, over time they will prove to be money well spent particularly for families with young children, the elderly and for those with allergies or poor health.

Another cause for concern is the modern architectural trend for building garages integral to the house. The problem here is the likelihood of various chemicals (solvents, pesticides, fungicides, varnishes, petrol tanks, oil cans, ageing paints and other volatile substances) being stored therein and the fumes emitted by such entering the house to the detriment of the householders. Ideally, all garages should be situated away from the home; if not, access should be arranged via an external door, in order to prevent noxious fumes from entering the living space. Wherever your garage is situated, ensure that the area is well ventilated at all times and that the number of stored substances is kept to an absolute minimum.

It is not just from chemical additives that we get toxic fumes: main appliances are frequently at fault, too. Poorly-maintained gas and oil-fired ovens, fires and boilers, as well as dirty chimney flues, can lead to the build-up of potentially fatal levels of carbon monoxide while being virtually unnoticed by the household. Simple-to-use detectors are readily available from hardware and plumbing shops but, in order to prevent problems arising, make sure that all such appliances are continuously and sufficiently well ventilated, kept clean, working correctly and regularly serviced. To minimize exposure further, choose an electric ignition rather than a pilot light and a boiler with a sealed combustion unit. Whenever the time comes to replace worn out appliances, ensure that the new one is energy efficient and installed by an engineer qualified to do so.

Electrical appliances and wiring also raise concerns as they give off radiation that causes a disturbance in the Earth's natural electromagnetic field. When at high levels, this electromagnetic stress is thought to impair the healthy functioning of the immune system and to contribute to conditions as diverse as insomnia, lethargy, joint pain and learning difficulties. Where possible, choose wooden-framed furniture and ensure that beds and sofas are situated away from walls that are adjacent to fuse boxes, air conditioning units or all-night electrical appliances such as refrigerators. Place sitting and sleeping positions away from cabling, switch appliances off at the plug and then remove the plug from the socket to reduce the risk further. In the bedroom, try to minimize the number of electrical appliances to one or two reading lamps and a battery-operated alarm clock. If you must use an electric clock, position it at least 4 feet from your head; having to get up to turn it off will make you get out of bed! Finally, replace your electric blanket with a hot water bottle to ensure warm feet and a truly undisturbed night's rest.

The presence of electrical equipment inside any enclosed space causes the negative ions in the atmosphere to become depleted. The now prevalent positive ions attract and hold dust particles in the atmosphere, causing irritation to the eyes and nose and throat. Using an ionizer will help to maintain the ratio of positive to negative ions, countering the effects of time spent around electrical appliances or in that modern day Faraday Cage, the car. By neutralizing the build-up of positive charge, the ionizer attracts not only dust out of the air but also smoke and pollen particles, too.

Along with ionizers, air filters and de-humidifiers also help to maintain a healthy atmosphere within the home, but do what you can to minimize the source of the problem. One of the biggest indoor pollutants is cigarette smoke; do yourself and your friends a favour and ban tobacco from the house. If someone insists on smoking in your home, put him or her by the open chimney or window and encourage them to exhale in that direction. Fortunately, one of the most efficient and decorative ways of getting rid of indoor pollutants is the presence of plants the best being ferns, palms, aloe vera, ficus trees and philodendrons. They also help to modify excess humidity. Combined with their beauty, energy and implicit invitation to nurture, this makes plants a vital component of any healthy home.

CHAPTER 4

Cleaning Up Your Home the Chemical-free Way

Over the years, our society has become more and more obsessed with the idea of living in a germ-free, clinically-sanitized environment. This obsession has been encouraged by the chemical industry, to the point where the average home is now full of manmade chemicals, all professing to protect us against naturally-occurring foreign bodies such as bacteria and germs. However, it was exposure to these natural antagonists throughout the course of our evolution that allowed our immune systems to develop sophisticated strategies for dealing with them, thereby facilitating the survival of the species. Many of the health problems that are manifesting today are a result of the sudden and enormous burden of new and highly-toxic chemicals that are being unleashed into our homes and straight into our bodies. Our beleaguered species faces the double whammy of under-exposure to the naturally occurring antigens needed for immune system development and, at the same time, bombardment by the noxious chemicals now found in everyday household products.

The reality is that many of the products sold to ensure our whiter-than-white lifestyles are made from the very dirtiest of ingredients. The fact that many of these substances are now sold in the form of a spray increases the likelihood of their causing damage, as the tiny airborne droplets can be inhaled directly into our lungs and so into our bloodstream. Whether they are absorbed through the skin or the respiratory tract, the toxicity of these chemicals is well-researched and well-documented, yet rarely do the warnings attached to these products accurately reflect their potential for harm. On the contrary, they are actively promoted as being health-supporting, a point particularly pressed home with the arrival of children. The mania for squeaky-clean cleanliness can easily be satisfied through the use of hot, soapy water and the implementation of basic standards of hygiene. Yet instead we are encouraged to use commercial disinfectants which are effectively pesticides known to the scientific community as being irritating to the skin as well as damaging to the respiratory tract if inhaled. Phenol (also known as carbolic acid) is the active ingredient in many cleaning products but the Material Safety Data Sheet that accompanies its production warns of its corrosive effects on the skin and, if inhaled (as can happen if sprays are used), its ability to burn the respiratory tract and cause gastric pain and nausea. Furthermore, as it is known to depress neurological functioning, damage can go on occurring for some time before the nerves register any pain.

Added to this are: solvents such as butyl cellosolve which, if inhaled or absorbed through the skin, can harm the central nervous system, the liver, the kidneys and the lymphatic system; detergents and surfactants that not only contain potentially carcinogenic substances but, when mixed with other chemicals, form carcinogenic nitrosamines which are readily absorbed through the skin; toilet cleaners containing paradichlorobenzene (a known irritant to the eyes, skin and mucus membranes) and naphthalene which carries the potential to inflict serious damage to the skin, liver and kidneys. Even more insidiously, there are chemicals which are hidden in seemingly innocuous products as a way of off-loading potentially expensive hazardous waste. Propylene, a form of toxic waste generated by the petroleum industry, is routinely incorporated into laundry detergent. In order to hide its nasty nature, it first has to be mixed with benzene to produce sulphuric acid, which then has to be neutralized by the addition of sodium hydroxide. To this is then added a sodium salt that resembles soap, all in order to create a product that can be marketed as soap. What with the carcinogens in your fabric softener and the neuro-toxins in your cleaning products, it really does seem as if we are more at risk inside our homes than out.

Just at the very time when our lives are becoming increasingly stressful, these chemicals are impairing the normal, healthy functioning of our immune systems. When our immune systems are impaired by excessive toxicity, they are less able to cope with the many naturally-occurring pathogens that life inevitably throws up. So, between the toxic stresses we introduce, the environmental stresses we encounter and the emotional stresses we have created, it's no wonder that we as a species are beginning to fail under the pressure of it all.

One simple and immediately effective way in which to reduce the likelihood of ill health is to lower the chemical load that our bodies are expected to carry. Perfectly adequate levels of hygiene can be achieved without recourse to hazardous chemicals or expensive outlay, thus ensuring the protection of both our homes and our family's health. Let us re-assess our attitude towards cleanliness within the home, throw out the synthetic chemicals and re-introduce some of the old and valid ways of keeping house, re-connecting ourselves to the wisdom of our grandmothers, lifting our spirits and supporting our health.

Note: although the following preparations use natural substances, it is nevertheless advisable to wear rubber gloves for heavier cleaning.

ESSENTIAL HELP

Essential oils will deodorize and disinfect your home and provide natural antibacterial action where needed. Make sure that they are stored safely, out of reach of children, and do not use them neat on the skin. A small bottle will last a long time; the following oils have been chosen for their price as well as their effectiveness. Place two drops on a cloth and wipe over or use eight drops in a 600ml-plant sprayer. Choose the citrus oils for effective action, without leaving a dominant smell. Use the stronger, herbal oils for floors, bins and heavier cleaning.

To disinfect & prevent bacterial growth:

- Lemon
- Lavender
- Pine
- Tea tree

To deodorize:

- Lime
- Orange
- Grapefruit
- Lemon

THE KITCHEN

SINKS, WORKTOPS AND REFRIGERATORS: mix one or two drops of one of the citrus essential oils listed above with hot water and a dash of vegetable-based detergent to hygienically wipe down the sink, fridge or work surface. Dry baking soda can be used as a scouring powder.

THE REFRIGERATOR: place a piece of charcoal in the larder, fridge or freezer to keep odours at bay. Change every few months. Keep the coils on the back of your refrigerator dust-free in order to maximize energy efficiency.

THE OVEN: for heavier cleaning, mix baking soda and water to form a paste and spread over the area. Leave for several minutes to allow it to lift grease effortlessly from the interior of your oven. For the toughest spots, use 1 tsp washing soda mixed with 2 tbsp distilled white vinegar, 1 tsp vegetable-based detergent and two cups of hot water and apply in the same way.

KITCHEN FLOORS: mix washing soda crystals in water for cleaning all non-wood or non-carpeted floors. Add essential oils as above to the final rinse water.

DRAINS: washing soda crystals will dissolve the greasy build-up that can contribute to blocked drains. For stubborn blockages, natural enzyme products are available.

Emptying the bin regularly, relocating the cat litter outside and ensuring that the dogs' blankets are kept clean will further reduce odours.

DE-SCALING: vinegar makes a very effective de-scaling agent. For the kettle, fill it half full (no more) with a mix of 50% vinegar and 50% water and boil up. It may require more than one treatment. Place a seashell inside to prevent further build up.

TO BANISH INSECTS AND MICE: to banish insects, place a few drops of lavender, peppermint or citronella essential oil on strips of ribbon and hang at open windows and doors to discourage insects from entering. To banish mice, mix a tablespoon of alcohol with 15 drops of peppermint oil and use it to soak some cotton wool. Place at access points around the house to deter entry. If necessary, humane traps are readily available; the caught mice can then be released unharmed into a natural habitat. Use peanut butter as bait.

THE SITTING ROOM

WINDOWS: use warm, soapy water and then rinse with a water and vinegar mix. Clean off with a wiper and polish with a scrunched-up newspaper.

DAMP DUSTING: mix a splash of vinegar in warm water to remove greasy marks from wood (not advised on high gloss finishes).

POLISH: many natural polishes made from beeswax and natural soap products are available.

BURNS ON CARPET: rub area with a cut potato immediately to minimize damage. Snip away scorch marks with scissors.

AIR FRESHENERS: opening the windows for just a few minutes will provide a complete change of air. Use a plant sprayer to freshen the air by adding to water a few drops of the deodorizing oils listed above.

THE BATHROOM

GENERAL CLEANING: add a few drops of lemon or pine essential oil to ordinary, vegetable-based detergent to hygienically clean the toilet, sink and bath. For scouring, use bicarbonate of soda. Invest in a good toilet brush with bristles all round and a holder that allows the bush to dry between uses.

LIME-SCALE BUILD-UP ON BATH AND TOILET: mix salt and hot vinegar into a paste and rub on the area using an old toothbrush. (Do not use metal, as it will scratch the surface.) For inside the toilet bowl, pour in one cup of vinegar and one tablespoon of baking soda and leave to effervesce for 15 minutes before flushing whilst scrubbing.

RUST MARKS ON BATH: mix salt, lemon juice and borax (from the chemist) into the stain and leave as long as necessary until bleached out.

THE BEDROOM

MOTH REPELLENT: string up chestnuts to deter moths. Make lavender sachets or use the oil on a piece of cotton wool.

FUNGUS AND MOULD ON WINDOWS: can generally be scrubbed off with an old toothbrush. Applying neat vinegar or tea tree oil will inhibit its return. Installing a trickle vent in the window unit will ensure continuous ventilation thereby reducing condensation.

THE LAUNDRY

Use only vegetable-based, eco-friendly washing liquids or detergents. Use the correct amount and always do a full load. Borax and washing soda can remove heavy stains. The Sun and the full Moon are both excellent bleaching agents; both are free and without environmental drawbacks. Line-dry clothes whenever possible.

❀ ❀ ❀   Beauty and the Beast   ❀ ❀ ❀

As has been seen, our homes are full of toxic cleaning substances that can easily and adequately be replaced by natural methods. However, equally toxic substances are also routinely included in the products designed to keep ourselves, our children and our pets clean: products which are acknowledged by the manufacturers themselves to cause liver, lung, brain, kidney and heart damage, as well as contact dermatitis, irritation of the mucus membranes and changes in skin cell formation. Yet we are encouraged to slather these substances over ourselves on a daily basis in the name of personal care and beauty. Why? Because these substances are relatively cheap and are therefore profitable. Of course, treatment of the increasing incidence of skin, mouth and throat cancers isn't cheap. Nor is the care involved in helping those whose internal organs have been damaged by the use of these products. But then that's not the problem of the chemical dealers. It's *our* problem, not just because ever more of our money is needed to support a struggling public health system, but because in the end we pay with our most valuable possession of all: our health.

The packaging on commercial toothpaste, for example, carries guidelines for usage but fails to make clear the risks associated with the long-term use of the substances contained within. One such substance is fluoride, an ingredient which most consumers would expect to see included as we are told that it protects our teeth. Historically, the reason for this was that researchers discovered that communities whose drinking water was high in naturally-occurring calcium fluoride had very few dental problems, leading them to believe that the addition of fluoride to toothpaste and water would benefit all. But, unfortunately for the general public, the fluorides routinely put in water and most toothpaste are not *calcium* fluoride but *silico*-fluorides the similarly-named but highly toxic by-products of industrial processes including aluminium production, nerve gas development and chemical fertilizer manufacture. The same product that is used in rat poison to grind up the intestines of rats is also recommended for our dental health.

The scientific tests used to declare that these silico-fluorides were not only safe but that they indeed helped to prevent tooth decay must have been severely flawed. For it is now known that, whereas calcium fluoride is only taken up by the body in minute doses, silico-fluorides are rapidly and readily absorbed (even when not swallowed) and are up to 85 times more toxic.

For the last 60 years, silico-fluorides have gone into the water supply of large areas of the population, into toothpaste, even into some milk and juice drinks for children. Only now is the truth of the matter coming to light. Incidence of fluorosis (where the teeth become pitted and discoloured) is increasing and over-exposure to silico-fluoride is now being linked to bone and tooth decay (including arthritis and osteoporosis), Alzheimer's Disease, memory loss, neurological impairment, kidney damage, bone cancer, increased incidence of fractures, genetic damage and stomach problems. Furthermore, it has been found to encourage the leaching of lead from old pipes, thus increasing our levels of lead absorption. Once again, substances presumed to be safe are in fact causing us serious health problems and, once again, it is only by becoming aware of the chemical reality behind the high-street hype that choices can be made about personal care which are more beauty than beast.

One of the most commonly-used substances is Sodium Lauryl Sulphate (SLS). This strong irritant is cheap and is used to produce the large quantities of foam we have come to (wrongly) associate with cleaning power. For this reason, it is present in nearly all mainstream personal care products: shampoo, toothpaste, face and body wash, bubble-bath, baby cleansers as well as in agent orange, garage floor cleaners and engine de-greasers. The Material Safety Data Sheet which accompanies SLS insists on the wearing of protective clothing, safety goggles, self-contained breathing apparatus and to ensure absolutely no contact with skin and eyes, nor inhalation or ingestion.

The scientific community recognizes SLS as a skin irritant, known to cause burning sensations in the mouth, shortness of breath, nausea and vomiting, which is the very reason why they use it to irritate the nasal and throat passages of the animals upon which they experiment. SLS is rapidly absorbed and retained in the tissues of the eyes, brain, heart, lungs and liver, causing both short- and long-term health problems. Furthermore, it is acknowledged that with both SLS and its alcohol form sodium laureth sulphate, there is a potential for carcinogenic formations of nitrates and dioxins when combined with the wide variety of other chemicals present in our personal care range. Yet they are still sold, without any declaration or warning, to be massaged into the scalp, skin and gums of the unwary public.

Added to this toxic cocktail are the chemicals found in many high-street beauty products. Glycerin is a common ingredient in moisturizers and so-called anti-ageing creams. The trouble is, unless you are in a high-humidity environment (which most of us are not), what glycerin actually does is draw moisture from the lower layers of the skin and hold it on the surface. Your skin may temporarily look better and feel smoother but you're actually hastening the ageing process. Ever wondered why men seem to age better than women? It is because they aren't obsessed with smothering these ageing creams on their faces?

Propylene glycol is another substance often included in formulations which are intended to feel smooth on the skin. In fact, it is a refined form of the oil used in automatic brake and hydraulic fluid. Along with all other mineral oils, it forms a filmy coating which suffocates the skin, preventing it from respiring naturally. As the skin is the body's largest excretory organ, impairing its ability to get rid of toxins means impairing our ability to remain healthy. The Material Safety Data sheets attached to propylene glycol acknowledge this through their warning that it is a known skin irritant and that its use carries the possibility of exacerbating kidney (an excretory organ) damage. The substances found in many antiperspirants have a similar effect, blocking the body's ability to rid itself of toxins and excess hormones, the efficient expulsion of which is crucial to our continuing good health.

Between the exfoliants known as Alpha Hydroxy Acids (AHAs), which in fact damage the skin's protective layer and the bentonite clay found in some cosmetic foundations, which causes pores to become clogged and the complexion to deteriorate, it can be very difficult to separate fact from fiction. The heady mix of supposedly scientific claims, newly-patented pseudo-scientific ingredients and airbrushed photos of women smiling strangely fixed smiles all serve to seduce us into believing the ad-men's hype, but hype is all it is. Personal care and beauty products rarely deliver on the promises they make; they frequently compromise our health while they are at it. The problems range from short-term flare-ups (such as contact dermatitis) to more serious and long-term organ damage. All of it is unnecessary and pointless.

Dr Michael Cork, head of Academic Dermatology at Sheffield University, recently published a study which looked at the incidence of eczema in young children.[2] Since the 1940s, incidence of this condition has increased dramatically; this rise perfectly coincides with our society's pattern of more frequent bathing and showering. Dr Cork and his colleagues found that the increased use of bathing products which has accompanied this change in lifestyle was one of the most important factors behind the increase in eczema. Many of the most well-known brands of bubble bath, soap, shower gel, shampoo and baby wipes contain crude surfactants, perfumes and, in some cases, even alcohol, all of which compromise the integrity of the skin. Dr Cork's report states that these substances break down the fats that occur naturally on the skin, disrupting the water content of the cells and so triggering the symptoms of eczema. His conclusion was that parents should treat eczema with prevention and simply avoid all conventional bathing products, replacing them with oil-based ones instead. The ingredients of conventional cleansers are known to cause skin problems. Yet the conclusions found by Dr Cork and other researchers seem to get lost beneath the onslaught of marketing campaigns that aim to convince you of their products' ability to create baby-soft skin: the very thing that your children had in the first place.

Are their alternatives? Happily, yes. A trip to your local health-food shop, one of the better supermarkets or a call to the right mail order company will demonstrate just what a range is available. You need to be vigilant as some of the products labelled 'natural' may still contain some of the harmful ingredients. However, having done some detective work and chosen the brands that fit your requirements, it simply becomes a matter of habit.

One step which you can easily take is to simplify your beauty routine and turn once again to nature for the answer. Beauty definitely comes from the inside and the best insurance against ageing comes in the form of proper nutrition, in particular the anti-oxidant vitamins A, C and E. Found in fruit and vegetables, these warrior vitamins are used by the body to dispose of the free radical particles and toxins that cause us literally to rust with age, making it far more sensible to invest your money in good, organic nutrition than in expensive, synthetic skin creams.

Secondly, drink water (non silico-fluoridated, of course) and plenty of it. Our bodies require at least eight glasses of water a day in order to maintain healthy functioning and even more during times of ill-health or recuperation. Unfortunately, we begin to dehydrate long before our bodies alert us to the problem and, because the brain's receptors for thirst and hunger are so closely associated, thirst is often mistaken for hunger and so left unquenched. The body treats fruit juice and fruit or herb teas as food, rather than water, so the daily quota needs to be drunk in addition to these. Regular tea and coffee act as diuretics, leaching more water from the body than they replace, thus incurring a further deficit that will again require topping up. Central heating and double-glazing further exacerbate the problem because they tend to lead to a very dry internal atmosphere, causing a loss of moisture from the skin. A lack of sufficient water also results in losses of important mineral salts such as potassium and sodium, needed by the heart, brain and kidneys to function healthily. Chronic dehydration is further implicated in constipation, backache, fatigue, joint pain, headaches, memory problems, Alzheimer's Disease and cancer. Unfortunately, the water arriving through our taps may contain traces of heavy metals, antibiotics, hormones, synthetic chemicals and even parasites. Furthermore, it tends to be very low in the organic minerals needed by the body. These are found in bottled water but, as this becomes expensive over a lifetime, a compromise can be reached by installing a good quality water filter, ideally fitted at the intake for the whole house, supplemented by a good quality, preferably liquid, mineral supplement. Sipped slowly and regularly throughout the day, water is one of the best health and beauty ensurers there is.

Sleep and relaxation are the other great aids to health and beauty. The amount of sleep needed varies from person to person, but make sure that you get what is adequate for you. If there simply aren't enough hours in the day (or night!) to get the sleep you need, try cultivating meditation techniques that, with practice, allow access to a deep and healing state where the mind is stilled and the body calmed. Exercise such as yoga or tai chi is another route to relaxation and, if you really can't find the energy for any of these, try at least to get a good massage. Above all, take the time to do what makes you happy because, when we feel happy and animated, our skin is plumped up by the increase in blood flow. This in turn helps to smooth out those wrinkles and makes our skin glow, doing away with the need for blusher. Our world as we experience it becomes literally etched on our faces: frown lines or laughter lines, tired eyes or sparkly ones. If we can learn to roll with life and resolve stress, we will be doing more for our looks than any injection of botox or collagen will ever do; after all, it is a physical impossibility to frown and laugh at the same time.

Finally, we can go back to the food cupboard which, again, provides a wealth of beauty-enhancing products. Pure vegetable oils (such as sweet almond) are absorbed into the skin, rather than sitting on top and blocking pores as the mineral oils do, making them a perfect base for cleansing as well as moisturizing. Oatmeal can be used for scrubs; eggs, honey or live yoghurt for face masks; cucumber for the eyes and the wonderful world of essential oils for just about everywhere. There are many books available which contain natural recipes for beauty but to get you started, here are some suggestions:

Facial scrub

Grind whatever pulses or nuts you have and mix with just enough sweet almond oil to moisten. Add 1 drop of essential oil of either cedarwood (to deep-cleanse an oily skin) or rosewood (to rejuvenate). Apply to the face and neck in a circular motion and then rinse off with splashes of cold water.

Face pack

- 1tbsp white (kaolin) clay
- tsp of cornflour
- 1 egg yolk
- 1tsp water
- 1 drop of *one* of the following essential oils:
- chamomile (for dry skin)
- rosemary (for oily skin)
- geranium (for combination skin)

Combine, apply and leave for twenty minutes before washing off with warm water.

Hand and body moisturizer

- 3 tbsp hazelnut or apricot kernel oil
- 1 tbsp hemp oil
- 4tbsp fragrant rose petals
- 8-10 drops geranium, rose or lavender essential oil
- 1tbsp beeswax granules
- Still spring water, warmed to approximately blood temperature

Place the oils in a *bain marie*. Heat until warm and then add the rose petals. Cover and leave for a minimum of four days. Sieve to remove the petals. Heat the beeswax in the bain marie, then blend in the rose-scented oil and the essential oils, stirring until the mixture cools. Beat in the water drop by drop until you achieve the consistency you require. Keep in a cool place and use as required.

Hair rinse

If blonde, use chamomile. Chamomile will not lighten the hair, but it is reputed to bring out the best in naturally blonde or fair hair. Make an infusion by pouring boiling water over the plant, while bruising it with a mortar or wooden spoon. Strain the mixture when cool and rub into the hair and roots after washing. Squeeze out the excess water and allow the hair to dry naturally. Refrigerate the remainder of the infusion for next time.

If brunette, use sage, rosemary and black China tea leaves. Make a strong infusion using a whole stem of sage, a whole stem of rosemary and a teaspoon of tea leaves. Apply as above.

Hairspray

Mix 1tsp of granulated sugar in a cup of warm water. Apply to damp hair. Dry and then lightly towel to soften the effect.

CHAPTER 6

What We Eat

The final area to address with regard to toxicity in the home is the food we eat. This is a scenario which has been getting progressively worse but, ironically, it began as a series of good intentions meant to ensure that Britain would never again face the food shortages it had experienced during the Second World War. It was this sudden vulnerability that caused a shell-shocked Britain to set up a system of intensive, subsidized farming intended to safeguard self-sufficiency in future times of crisis. Unfortunately, this understandable reaction soon mutated into an era of greed and environmental devastation that spread the world over. In place of the mixed farming practices of yesteryear, where knowledge of good husbandry, crop rotation, companion planting and the ethos of guardianship had successfully prevailed for generations, a new approach was masterminded by the chemical industry. In the rush to cash in on the massive increases in yield facilitated by the use of chemical additives such as fertilizers, pesticides, herbicides and fungicides, the majority of farmers and agricultural policy makers embraced this new development without ever questioning the long-term impact.

For example, since the 1950s farmers have been encouraged to use synthetic hormone weed-killers on crops and growth-promoting hormones on livestock. Now, as cancer rates soar and fertility rates plummet, we have to question the wisdom of ever introducing such potent and disruptive chemicals into our food chain. The dreaded DDT, once widely promoted as the answer to all humankind's insect-borne woes, was finally withdrawn but only after it had decimated the bird population and there are still un-quantifiable implications for future generations, such is its persistence in the food chain. Unfortunately, DDT and its fellow organochlorine pesticides were replaced by a whole new group of toxins called organophosphates (OPs) which, as well as killing off the warble fly as intended, have the effect of preventing nerve cells from connecting with one another. In his excellent book, *The Great Food Gamble*, John Humphrys notes that there is a higher incidence of cases of BSE in areas of high organophosphate use. He asks whether the increase in incidence of diseases such as Alzheimer's, Parkinson's, attention deficit disorders and, of course, vCJD could also be linked to the routine use of the organophosphates. Although no connection has ever been proven, we might bear in mind that there are very few financially independent scientists.

While the chemical corporations assure us of the rigorousness of their research, the fact is that almost all scientific research is commissioned and/or carried out by those with a vested interest in the outcome. Scientific research is itself a self-regulating industry worth billions of dollars.

The scientists themselves are generally bound by confidentiality agreements which prevent them from speaking out about any disclosure that may harm the project. As the research is often geared towards confirming whatever the commissioning company wants to promote, the possibility of goal-posts being moved and negative findings being buried becomes a real threat to honest disclosure. In fact, research misconduct (including overtly fraudulent manipulation of data) is such an acknowledged reality that in 1998 the editors of *The Lancet, The British Medical Journal* and *Gut* set up the Committee of Publication Ethics (COPE) to draw attention to this problem[3]. As COPE battles to ensure the integrity of any research that comes its way, its aim is to set up a code of practice for researchers and editors as well as for the universities, private companies and public health institutions which employ them.

As far as our food is concerned, the result of all this is that whilst successive governments have declared war on cancer, heart disease and other illnesses of the moment, they have continued to give their heartfelt approval to the practice of annually spraying millions of gallons of agricultural chemicals straight onto our food crops. The problems caused by these toxins are further exacerbated by the fact that the nutritional value of our food has plummeted to the point where its mineral and vitamin content is now a fraction of what it was before the industrialization of our food production.

Studies from the UK, the US and Canada all confirm a significant and often dramatic decrease in the nutrient levels now present in plant foods including iron, calcium, magnesium, potassium and copper, as well as in the important anti-oxidant vitamins A and C. So great has been the revolution in our food production methods that we now have crops grown hydroponically, i.e. without soil and suspended in a water solution enriched with a limited range of minerals. Fruit crops are often harvested before they are fully ripe, meaning that the plant will not have had time to fully develop the fruit's vitamin content. Nutrient levels are further compromised because crops are stored for far longer than would have previously been possible and they are grown in environments where water, air and soil quality is jeopardized by chemical pollution. But the most likely cause of this rapid nutritional devaluation of our food crops is that intensive farming relies on three main mineral additives: nitrogen, phosphorous and potassium in order to produce crops that not only appear to be healthy but can be grown repeatedly and in quick succession on the same patch of soil. Unfortunately, the repeated plantings facilitated by these additives leads to the soil's becoming depleted in the full spectrum of minerals and trace elements necessary for the proper, whole health of the plant. As a result, any human which then feeds on these nutrient-impoverished crops also becomes depleted in the very nutrients that ensured our successful journey to the top of the food chain.

Efforts are being made to add certain minerals artificially (either to the soil or to the finished food product) but the body's assimilation of these base elements is a precision-tuned balance: overdose on one and you severely impact on the body's ability to access another. The resulting depletion in our bodily stock of naturally-accessed resources means that, despite having year-round access to a wide range of fruit and vegetables, we have a chronically ill population.

Magnesium deficiency can result in arteriole rigidity and spasms; a lack of potassium to liver disease and impaired reflexes, and a severe depletion of calcium to arthritis and bone loss. Vitamin A is needed for the healthy growth and maintenance of body tissues, including the eyes. Vitamin C aids the absorption of iron, which is necessary for the health of our blood vessels, skin and gums. Vitamin E is needed for hormone production and for the health of our blood cells while all of these antioxidant vitamins are crucial to our ability to fight disease. Vitamin and mineral deficiency will always result in some form of ill health, yet modern intensive farming does nothing to ensure the health of the soil upon which we ultimately rely for nourishment. Instead, we invest in the attempt to cure the results of these deficiencies via our national health system; itself in a state of possibly terminal decline due to its own long-term deficiency: funding.

But the problem is not limited to fruit and vegetables. 'New' and 'improved' foodstuffs which have, in reality, been over-processed and messed about with to the point where they become injurious to our health are continually being marketed to the householder. The development of margarine is a classic example. Originally touted as the healthy, low-fat alternative to butter, it has since been discovered that the hydrogenation process involved in making margarine creates trans-fatty acids.

These have subsequently been acknowledged to have a hugely negative impact on the body's ability to utilize naturally-occurring essential fatty acids. However, this has not brought an end to the use of this process; hydrogenated fats are now found in everything from biscuits to cakes, fast food, convenience food, and even vegetarian options which are often presumed to be the healthier choice. The epidemic of heart disease now afflicting Western societies coincides with the wholesale acceptance of hydrogenated fats in our diet yet, despite this, we persist in believing what those guardians of our health tell us and continue to forsake good old natural (i.e. organic) butter for something resembling plastic.

For too long, government ministers have accepted wholesale and without question the information given to them by profit-motivated agrochemical companies whilst, at the same time, resisting assertions made by international health organizations and environmentalists regarding long-term ecological and health issues.

By passively accepting the advice given to them by the men from the Ministry, farmers have also made themselves culpable in this mess we call a food industry. But we consumers must also take our share of the responsibility, because by buying into the notion that cheap food is good food and that year-round availability and appearance is more important than nutritional value or even taste, we are culpable in the poisoning of both ourselves and the planet.

At a time when cookery shows are all the rage and chefs are celebrities, we have allowed ourselves to become nutritionally weakened to the point where our body's ability to organize health on a cellular level is being severely compromised. The natural intelligence that governs internal health also expresses itself through thought processes and actions, which is why animals know which grasses have medicinal properties without ever being taught and why birds know to migrate with the changing seasons. To us humans, this innate intelligence goes by the name of common sense and when we choose to leave it behind, breakdown inevitably ensues.

Investing in one's health begins by listening to innate good sense and this can only mean investing in good quality, organic, free range food, even if it costs a few pence more. Having woken up to the realities of modern food production, we must take the initiative and put our money literally where our mouths are. With companies who only understand profit, we, the consumer, become a very powerful lobby, but only if we choose to be so. These days, consumer power is much more effective than the political vote and capable of packing a far more direct punch. When the middle-class masses decided that they didn't want genetically-modified (GM) foods, many of the major supermarkets responded by immediately removing such products from their shelves, such is the power in our pocket.

It is imperative both for our own health and the health of the planet that we take on board the need to move towards a more organic-based future for food production. Although our soil will take time to recover, studies show that organically-grown food is indeed safer and better for us. The UK organic standards organisation, the Soil Association, states that on average organic food contains higher levels of vitamin C, magnesium, calcium, chromium and iron, as well as increased levels of antioxidants vitamins. Furthermore, because the standards set by the Soil Association demand that farmers avoid the 400-odd pesticides used in conventional farming, there is a greatly reduced risk of harmful residues reaching the customer. By prohibiting the use of GM crops, both for customers and as animal feed, organic farming methods provide a tried and tested alternative to the newly-touted and relatively (though terrifyingly) untested genetically-modified future. At a time when consumer confidence is being sorely tried, organic farming offers a common sense approach which does not need the dubious statistics relied upon by the chemical industry. It is wholly and conclusively backed by the hundreds of years of sustainable practice that preceded the chemical warfare now dominating our food supply (and therefore our health). If we the consumer demand it, the message that organic produce is a market to exploit will trickle through to the supermarket giants while politicians will realize that it is a vote winner. Only then, when all those chemical poisons have been removed from our food production, will we begin to see a return to health for both ourselves and our global home.

Fortunately, whilst we in the West languish in a nutritional abyss, more and more farmers in Africa, Asia and South and Central America are returning to more organically-based, mixed farming methods and by doing so are actually able to increase yields. Whilst the chemical giants insist that it is impossible to feed the world organically, farmers here found that increasing pest and disease immunity rendered the accumulating cost of pesticides prohibitive to their pockets and injurious to their health. They decided that they had no option but to turn their backs on the intensive practices of conventional farming and to return instead to the organic, mixed farming practices of their forefathers.

Having taken this brave step, they are now finding that yields have started to increase by as much as 175% and that costs are decreasing by as much as 30%. This somewhat surprising finding was documented in *The Real Green Revolution* report (February 2002)[4], by Nicholas Parrott and Terry Marsden of the Greenpeace Environmental Trust, and directly challenges the big players whose profits depend on our remaining chemically-dependent. The farmers are achieving these results by growing a variety of crops all year round and by using their understanding of the complexities of the natural ecosystem to inhibit unwanted pests and diseases. These production methods, which allow increased yields of nutritionally more valid crops, are further endorsed by lowered investment costs.

Just as these farmers reclaimed their land, their health and their profits from the clutches of the chemical-mongers, so we must reclaim our right to good, safe food. We must insist on it. For the whole of our evolution, food has been not only our fuel but our medicine also. The multi-billion dollar industries that include intensive farming, diet food, supplements and health-care all manage to obscure the same basic point: that what we need to maintain healthy bodily functioning is a balanced diet of nutritionally-viable foods. We are naturally designed to be healthy. We would not have survived the rigours of natural selection if we weren't. It is much simpler than the scientists would have us believe. Ultimately, it is down to us as individuals to decide what goes into our bodies. So, ignore the mystifying processes at large and go with innate intelligence. Go for good quality, organic food bought in season and give frequent reminders to the market managers and local shops that you'd like to see more.

CHAPTER 7

How We Eat

One of the least-appetizing marketing ploys of recent years has been the introduction and acceptance of what have become known as convenience foods. Quite why it was decided that a ritual as profoundly important to our wellbeing could, or should, ever be considered inconvenient is depressing to contemplate. The drive towards maximum productivity that dominated our food policies was mirrored in the workplace. Working hours increased, women were encouraged to break free from the shackles of the kitchen and our insatiable desire for having all things available at all times meant that shift work began to permeate our culture as the norm.

The result of this new thinking is that, where eating together had previously been as much a part of family life as all sleeping under the same roof, it has now been sidelined to the margins. As pressure on our time grew, these new so-called convenience meals were welcomed and the subtle implication that traditional cooking was somehow an inconvenience began to permeate our thinking. The 2005 British Lifestyles[5] report, by research company Mintel, found that the convenience foods sector now accounts for over 30% of all consumer spending on food. It states that, in 2004, UK consumers spent a staggering £12billion on pre-made meals, sweet and savoury snacks and puddings. On the other hand, primary foods such as meat and fish accounted for only a fifth of spending. Mintel's research predicts that the amount of 'convenience seekers' will grow as average household sizes continue to diminish.

The nutritional value of many of these processed foods with their high salt and fat contents, their trans-fatty acids and their dubious sources of protein is questionable to say the least but equally dangerous is the fact that these fast food alternatives completely ignore the ritual attached to the consumption of food.

From the order in which the pack/tribe ate, to the convoluted ceremonies of formal eating, food has always been used to nurture clan stability and reinforce social standing. The phrase 'the family that eats together stays together' is one that contains real wisdom and yet it seems as if this fundamental part of communal life has been subjected to a kind of time and motion study and somehow been found wanting. In fact, the provision and sharing of food is so entirely bound up with the flow of love that something quite magical occurs when family or friends sit down together for a freshly prepared meal and, as we shall see, the benefits go way beyond mere vitamins and minerals.

Our physical and mental response to every aspect of our life experience, including the consumption of food, begins in the brain. Our senses pick up environmental clues and send messages to the cerebrum to be analysed and acted upon. Before any thing even enters our mouths, our digestive processes are stimulated into action by the sights, smells and sounds of food preparation. Therefore, for our stomachs to be at an optimum state of readiness to receive food, some advanced warning is required, whether that be through choosing recipes, chopping vegetables, cooking or gathering together around a tantalizingly set table: all will stimulate the brain into anticipatory readiness. Food eaten without due attention i.e. on the run, whilst distracted by work or if distilled into the form of a drink is less likely to be recognized by the brain as having been eaten. This means that you are likely to feel hungry again sooner than if you fully engage your brain in the eating process; a point generally missed by the diet industry.

In preparing our bodies to receive food, it is also important to consider our stress levels around mealtimes. When stressed, the body produces adrenalin, a hormonal response which has the effect of inhibiting the digestive process. An inability to relax around mealtimes tends to lead to stagnation within the gut, which then has a serious impact on the body's ability to absorb nutrition. The toxicity which then results from all of this improperly digested food lies behind many of the most common health problems experienced today such as bloating, back ache, constipation and its sister act, diarrhoea. This tells us that the way in which we eat is just as important as the quality of the food that we choose to eat.

Finally, in order to understand fully the impact of stress on nutritional status, it is also necessary to question the impact of stress on the foodstuff itself. Japanese scientist Masaru Emoto developed a technique for photographing frozen water crystals, which he then recorded and analysed. In doing so, he revealed that the formation of each crystal was affected by the conditions to which it was exposed. The results recorded in his book, *Messages from Water, Vol.1*, are truly astonishing, as the crystals appear to take on different characteristics according to their experiences. As one might expect, crystals from a mountain spring appear as perfect snowflakes whereas ones from polluted urban waters are almost unrecognizable, in some cases prevented from developing any form of crystalline structure on account of contamination. But Dr Emoto goes further, taking phials of water from the same source and then introducing different vibratory influences, such as classical as opposed to aggressive rock music, or words of kindness and encouragement as opposed to those that imply anger or hostility. Amazingly, the photographs show how the water crystals appear to capture and then reflect back the sense of these words and music. His exquisite photographs show that positive vibrations can be used to positively enhance the quality of the crystals, therefore revealing water to be a potential tool for healing the plants, animals and humans who then drink it.

His findings further indicate the possibility that the water molecules contained within our physical bodies, as well as all that comprise our planetary home, will be resonating with the vibrations of our emotions, thoughts and actions. When we feel angry, we carry the resonance of those angry thoughts, words and deeds in the very waters of our bodies. We truly do ourselves harm by the thoughts which we harbour, reaping precisely that which we sow.

This is a very sobering thought, but at the same time it is truly inspirational. Think what can manifest through thoughts that are kind, compassionate and empathetic. Think of the potential for self-harm or self-healing that this offers. Think, then, of animals raised in pain and killed in fear. Think of how their suffering becomes recorded in the very essence of their cells. Think of the meat you eat. Being a part of the food chain is a natural part of life but the gross exploitation of defenceless animals for cheap meat and fat profit is outside nature and debases humanity. The case for humane farming practices again becomes paramount. If you wish to eat meat, insist on strict animal welfare standards; once again, that will mean free range, organic produce only.

The final gift that water has to offer is the chance of redemption for, as Dr Emoto's work reveals, prayer and meditation have the power to bring healing to troubled waters. By honouring the food that we eat, with sincere gratitude for the sacrifice and care involved in its provision, it is perhaps possible to enhance the very structure of the water molecules within it and so access healing. At one time, the saying of Grace was part of every meal but today the ritual of giving thanks before taking food has largely been forgotten. When preparing to take nourishment, a prayer of thanks either to your god or to the benevolent Earth will create a harmonizing link between yourself and the wider natural world and provides a wonderful example of the clear link between good spiritual practice and good physical health.

Directing practical, mental and spiritual focus towards the food we eat greatly enhances the benefit we receive from it: investing in organic farming methods with their high standards of animal care; taking the time to prepare vibrant, tasty food; ensuring the quietude necessary for obtaining all the nourishment we need and by eating together with a sense of grace and gratitude, we provide the firm foundation from which our physical health can be built.

CHAPTER 8

How We Recognize and Resolve Physical Discomfort

Having rid our homes of chemical blight and filled our cupboards instead with safe, natural alternatives, we can now begin to assess how much physical comfort is provided by the home and whether there is anything that can be done to improve matters. All sorts of physical problems, from backaches to headaches to ligament stress, are caused simply by ill-suited, inappropriately placed or poorly-designed furniture and appliances. Back problems account for huge losses in industrial and corporate output and employers are beginning to recognize the benefits of looking after the backs of their workforce. In the home, we too can ensure the health of our skeletal and muscular systems by taking the time to modify or install designs that suit our physical needs. Obviously, most items of furniture are going to be used at one time or another by people of varying ages and sizes but there are some general guidelines available.

Ascertaining how efficiently people are able to operate in a given environment is known as ergonomic assessment and this information can be used to find ways of reducing muscular stress and general fatigue, thereby improving performance. As the kitchen is the hardest-working of all the rooms in the house, it makes a logical starting point for such an appraisal.

If you are designing your kitchen from scratch, it is important to ensure that the three main stations (the sink, the fridge and the cooker) are within easy reach of each other, otherwise the cook will become exhausted with all the unnecessary to-ing and fro-ing. To avoid this, position these three primary appliances in a proportionately-spaced triangle or alternatively, follow an uninterrupted line, L- or U-shape interposed with adequate work surfaces. Whether the main user is left- or right-handed will also make a difference to the layout, as a right-handed person will tend to proceed from left to right, i.e. from sink to drainer to surface to further appliance and so on. If the main user is left-handed, the ideal layout will be the reverse of this. However, remember that at some point you may wish to sell your home and the chances are that it will be to a right-handed person. The compromise is to install a sink with a drainer on both sides and to ensure adequate work surfaces on either side of the cooker. As a further point of design, try to ensure the absence of through traffic, which can be hazardous when full pots and pans are being moved about.

Next, think about heights and surface levels as the difference of a few centimetres can render a task truly backbreaking. The optimal height for a work surface is about 100mm below elbow level, whose elbow depends on who the main user is! Most of us have backs that can put up with a little discomfort but, if your back is vulnerable, getting the surface height right will be an excellent long-term investment. If you are particularly tall, free-standing units offer a solution as these can be raised on blocks which can later be removed for the purposes of selling without causing problems for the wall tiles.

Some so-called time-saving appliances can be very wearing on the body and none more so than the dishwasher. Bending and twisting while carrying heavy crockery can be very injurious to backs and, as older models often require the rinsing or soaking of dishes prior to the machine being switched on, their real value is questionable. Low-level grills are another appliance that require us to bend at awkward angles whilst simultaneously handling weighted grill pans, so if your back is vulnerable go for an eye-level one instead. Combined fridge/freezers are now commonplace and space-saving, but always ensure that it is the fridge (which is used most often) that occupies the top half of the appliance for ease of access.

When choosing either appliances or cupboards, consider how easy particular designs are going to be to keep clean. Surfaces with lots of nooks and crannies are much harder to keep dust and grease free and so will, again, incur physical cost to you.

On the subject of cupboards, take the time to assess your storage needs. The reason work surfaces tend to get cluttered is that they provide the most accessible storage facility. Most cupboard space has little optimal storage, the majority being difficult to reach places like right at the back, too high up or too deep to reach in without moving the stuff in front. Deep cupboards, particularly deep, high cupboards are not the solutions that they appear to be. Count yourself very lucky if you happen to own a real, walk-in larder as these provide the best food storage of all. As a final thought, question how much cupboard space is really necessary. You'll fill whatever you have, so think about just how many gadgets, sets of china, cookery books and so on you really need.

After a hard day everyone needs a good night's sleep and a good bed is the best way to achieve it. For a long time, a hard mattress was said to benefit tired backs. However, this advice has since been revised and now the recommendation is for a multi-sprung mattress that allows for a suitable degree of give. This give allows the mattress to support the body in the wide variety of postures adopted throughout an average night's sleep, thus helping to avoid the build-up of muscular tension and pressure on joints which may otherwise cause us to wake. Of course, the bed should also be wide enough and long enough to accommodate any nightly fidgets without causing oneself or one's sleeping partner any problems.

Workstations are another area where the body is expected to work hard. As more and more people opt to work from home, it is important to invest in the best quality support for your back that you can afford. Again, the aim is to limit muscular and ligament stress, reduce the impact of compressive force on the lower region of the spine and to allow free circulation of blood and lymph.

Begin by ensuring that your office chair is as fully adjustable as possible. Find a seat which is firm but padded and covered in material that is porous (to allow ventilation) and rough in texture (to prevent slipping). Ideally, the seat height should come to fractionally below the back of the knee. In order for it to feel at an appropriate level with the table, it may be necessary to have a higher seat, in which case a footrest can be improvised. The seat should ideally reach from the back of the buttock to just before the knee: too deep and it will increase pressure on the back of the knee, impairing the flow of blood and lymph. The backrest should have a moulded shape in order to give adequate support to the concave curve of the lower spine. If this is absent, a pillow may be placed in the small of the back instead. Above the lumbar region, a very gentle concave curve in the backrest is acceptable, but flat is preferable to over-pronounced. A reclining back-tilt at an angle of approximately 95-100 degrees to the seat will provide a compromise between reducing the compressive force between trunk and hips without increasing the horizontal force to the point of forcing the buttock forward. This tilt is advisable with a medium-to-high backrest only, otherwise the body becomes unstable. At the same time, the seat can be tilted up by approximately 5 degrees in order to minimize the tendency to slip forwards.

Armrests add support and aid standing but they should be well padded to reduce any trauma to the delicate area under the wrist and forearm. (If armrests are unpadded or simply not present, wrist pads can be worn to protect the wrists as they hit the desk.) Armrests should not interfere with the desk and should be low enough to allow the upper arms to hang loosely, so as not to cause a hunching of the shoulder. Keep the area under the desk as clear of clutter as possible.

Ensure that the desk allows the computer monitor to be between 500mm and 750mm from your eyes. The monitor should be of adequate size, with a high quality image. Centre the screen a little below eye level at an angle of approximately 15 degrees. Keep it at right angles to any windows and try to ensure that no lighting is reflected onto the screen. If you habitually work from documents, invest in document holders placed at a similar height to the screen, or between the keyboard and screen, in order to minimize neck-turning and fatigue.

Obviously, most chairs within the home are for more relaxed sitting; however, the principles are much the same. For comfy seating, such as the sofa or armchairs, ensure adequate back height to support the upper back, shoulders and neck and provide a scattering of cushions for extra lumbar support. The provision of a footstool will make your seating appropriate for a wider variety of user sizes and hopefully encourage the blood to keep flowing through out-stretched legs rather than having to squeeze through tucked-up ones. If mobility is a problem, make sure that your comfy chairs are not so low as to make standing difficult. Again, as with an office chair, ensure that your dining chairs provide adequate backrests, a seat depth that does not interfere with blood flow and a seat height that does not elicit a tendency to slip forward. As with all aspects of day-to-day life, your dinner parties will be far more enjoyable if everyone is sitting comfortably.

❀ ❀ ❀   Ease and Dis-ease   ❀ ❀ ❀

Although spring cleaning is a term often used in reference to the house, it can also be used in reference to our own physical home: ourselves. As we all know, clearing out cupboards and sweeping through the house lifts the spirits immeasurably, but what's less well understood is that this, or any physical action, stimulates the lymphatic system which is itself the cleansing system of the body. By keeping our lymphatic system moving, we help it to do its job of filtering out unwanted by-products, such as pre-cancerous cells, free radical particles and those implicated in heart disease. A healthy, active body is very efficient at this process; even so, it is vital to our long-term health that we stop and recognize any feelings of dis-ease, dis-comfort or dis-stress as and when they arise. Pain is nature's way of telling us that something is wrong, either physically or emotionally, and the sooner it is acknowledged, the sooner our healing can begin.

Early warning signs that a body is under physical or emotional stress include the following: tiredness, lethargy, impaired memory, irritable bowel, susceptibility to viral infections, non-specific aches and pains, tension headaches, irrational eating patterns, irritability and insomnia. To help us cope with stress, the body releases powerful painkillers; often vital in the short-term, if the stress persists then these hormones can blunt the internal messages which our bodies are sending us. Unfortunately, society encourages us not to acknowledge these early warning signs; taking time out is not permitted until we actually fall measurably ill, at which point the drug industry is there to ensure that we are back out in the market place as soon as possible. But in the long term, it is our ability to understand the true nature of dis-ease that ultimately determines our success at preventing it, allowing us instead to maintain holistic health.

The Western approach to medicine has involved the mapping, dissection, analysis and theorization of the human body for centuries, yet we still seem no closer to our goal of good health into old age. The allopathic system of health which dominates Western medical practice today addresses disease by counteracting the manifestations or symptoms of any given illness, mainly through the use of surgical procedures and synthetic drugs. By definition, what it doesn't do is address what's causing the illness in the first place. This is very fortunate for those in the business of producing symptom-suppressing drugs as, obviously, there is little or no profit to be made in actually curing people. Rather than effecting a cure, most drugs simply allow people to cope with their illness, possibly stopping it from progressing but invariably setting off a whole series of side-effects which the body then has to cope with in addition to the initial illness. Over-the-counter painkillers are a prime example of how we are encouraged to ignore our body's own wisdom on the advice of those who make vast profits out of our continued ignorance. Whilst no-one would wish to deny a seriously ill patient relief from their physical pain, if we were less ready to use painkillers to mask our discomfort in the first place, many illnesses could be addressed before they get out of control. Persistent headaches, for instance, may indicate anything from high blood-pressure to stress to allergy to brain tumour; how are we to begin healing if we simply blunt our feeling and continue to deny what our bodies are trying to tell us?

Despite years of scientific research, our bodies still retain their fundamental mystery. However, as the Western approach to life and health continues to throw up problems, people are turning to alternatives and doctors are having to take note. In some corners of medical thinking, a shift is beginning to occur acknowledging that, until the role of the mind in bodily welfare is recognized, the true nature of ill health will never be fully understood. One of the most fascinating areas of investigation into the mind/body connection involves the use of placebos.

Placebos are essentially dummy pills which are given to patients who believe them to be the real thing. The placebo effect of mind over body is so strong that patients receiving these pills have initiated the healing of everything from backache to stomach ulcers. Many of the drugs developed to combat physical symptoms are subsequently withdrawn, having been found to be only as effective (or even less so) as placebos. From allergy vaccines to antidepressants, trials using placebos have shown that the benefits supposedly obtained by using drugs actually come from the patients' belief that things would improve, rather than the action of the drug itself. Yet synthetic drugs are still prescribed and imbibed, despite acknowledged side-effects which can include palpitations, visual blurring, tremors, diarrhoea, rashes, loss of sex drive, cataracts, glaucoma, stomach bleeding, organ damage, arthritis and more. Nor is it just allergic reactions and depression that can find relief through belief: anxiety, angina, heart disease and even cancer are all significantly influenced by our mindset. Fake operations have given benefit to sufferers of diseases as diverse as Parkinson's and arthritis and fake analgesics have been shown to initiate the patient's own pain-relieving mechanisms.

It is well known that patients fare far better if they feel supported and listened to, but many time-pressured consultants and registrars seem more ready to treat symptoms than humans, happier to quote probable outcomes than possible ones. Such negative influences have an equally powerful impact on our expectations and the subsequent outcome. Known as a nocebo, this negative effect lies behind many of the stories of witchcraft, voodoo and spell-making to be found around the world. If you believe strongly enough in the power of the hex be it a pill, a potion, a prognosis or an enchantment, whether for good or bad, your body will initiate all the complex molecular changes required to manifest the prescribed outcome. The placebo/nocebo phenomenon is one that terrifies many doctors to the point where they simply deny it or become alarmist at the prospect of a return to the age of faith healers, quacks and old wives' tales. And yet the alternative which they offer is one that relies on chemicals toxic to our bodies and techniques so invasive that they carry huge risks.

Our continuing trust in our doctors and the pharmaceutical giants who supply them is more the result of a successful marketing campaign and social pressure than with empirical evidence. Steve Ransom, research director at Credence Publications, states that the worldwide conventional cancer drug market is expected to exceed $27 billion by 2005. In his book, *Great News on Cancer in the 21st Century* (Credence), he argues that the true war on cancer is about politics and the protection of a multi-billion dollar industry. He lists many examples of viable, health-supporting alternatives (backed up by credible research) that have been sidelined, distorted and suppressed by a powerful and greedy pharmaceutical industry more interested in profit margins than in people's lives.

This manipulation of the truth regarding our health and ability to heal has been exacerbated by the fact that we, as a society, simply do not expect to have to take responsibility for our own wellbeing, either financially or spiritually. Since the advent of the National Health Service, the majority of people have happily allowed others to be in charge of their health, relying increasingly on prescription pills to blunt physical and emotional suffering instead of listening to the messages encoded in that pain. Yet, as the placebo phenomenon shows, we have the ability to respond effectively to pain and to initiate our own healing simply by choosing to do so at a very deep level in our consciousness. By making changes at the deepest level of our being, in our beliefs and expectations, we can open the channel for communication between mind and body; this is the key to attaining real, holistic health. For this to happen, it is essential that we feel secure and supported enough to trust our own inner voice. The next section therefore explores the role of the home as a primary emotional support, the perfect antidote to the stresses of modern survival.

Section 2

THE EMOTIONAL
HOME

CHAPTER 10

Creating Health

While some of the benefits secured by a non-toxic, physically supportive home become apparent over the long term, others are more immediate. It may take the whole summer to discover that, having banished synthetically-fragranced cleaning products your seasonal sniffles are less problematic, but as soon as you make the decision to buy chemical-free, body-friendly products something very profound will take place. Your whole being will physiologically respond to the good feeling that such life-affirming actions give you. As your hormonal system sighs with happiness, so your internal equilibrium is restored and maintained. It is the maintenance of this harmonious balance that is the key to holistic health.

At last, our society is beginning to re-acknowledge the notion that emotional happiness can influence physical wellbeing. But for the last several hundred years, we have been encouraged to view mind and body as separately-functioning entities and it was this thinking that led to the splitting of our psychological and physiological selves. The process began during the Middle Ages when the prevailing religious doctrine of Northern Europe decreed that the needs of the physical body should be repressed and that only the spiritual self be tended and glorified. Later, as the influence of religion receded and the age of scientific discovery flourished, the physical anatomy and physiology of our bodies was brought into focus and fuelled a new obsession with the 'how' rather than the 'why'.

It is only relatively recently that the link between mind and body has begun to be re-examined. In the 1960s, pioneers in the fields of personal development, healing and alternative health began to bring back skills and knowledge acquired in the East in order to radically re-interpret what constituted holistic health. This new approach was ready to view our physical state as a manifestation of our internal emotional state, which meant that practitioners now worked on both the physical and emotional level in order to effect whole body healing. The innate good sense of this approach is obvious once it is accepted that, without changes in our approach to life through diet, exercise, attitude or expectation, any medical intervention can only be of a sticking-plaster nature.

The mind/body connection is made physiologically through the actions of our nervous and hormonal systems. The somatic division of the peripheral nervous system (PNS) picks up messages regarding the outside world, which are then sent to the brain. Depending on what action the brain decides upon, messages are then relayed via the central nervous system to the autonomic division of the PNS, which is concerned with the subconscious regulation of internal activity including the release or inhibition of hormones, heart rate, internal temperature and so on. Depending on the brain's interpretation of the initial message, the autonomic system will initiate either the *sympathetic* pathway of reaction, which activates the stress responses and prepares the body to flee, fight or freeze or, alternatively, the *parasympathetic* reaction, which acts to conserve energy or restore equilibrium. This means that our two basic responses to any given stimulus are either to react or to relax.

It is a strange indictment of our psyches that it is often easier to accept this mind/body connection when it is seen in the negative. For example, if the driver in front of us is driving particularly slowly, we may well experience the following effects: the adoption of a more aggressive posture, a rise in blood pressure and increased heart rate. All of these are physiological reactions to an emotional crisis. We have not been hurt or confronted but we are required to make a mental choice between a) driving more slowly ourselves or b) risking overtaking. This then requires further mental processing before we put our final decision in to practice physically. Do we relax or do we react? It is the choices made at moments like these that ultimately define our state of health.

Although the physical discomfort that arises from such emotional disturbances is very real, it should be remembered that emotional stress is the mental anticipation of an event, not the event itself. If we see someone coming towards us with a knife and we believe that they may harm us, our stress response comes into effect via the actions of the sympathetic nervous system and we prepare for fight or flight or we simply freeze with terror. Our subconscious, physiological response to this mental appraisal of the situation is to re-route blood away from the body's surface, hence we go white with fear. This allows us to conserve blood in the event of wounding, and directs it instead towards the muscles in order to increase our ability to run or fight more efficiently. Our heartbeat increases to maintain this supply, whilst our bronchial tubes dilate to increase the amount of oxygen available. Our digestive processes are inhibited and, in cases of acute anxiety, the system will spontaneously empty. Our pupils dilate, allowing us to take in more light and we begin to sweat in order to ensure that our bodies remain cool in the face of increased exertion. Our liver begins to breakdown glycogen to meet the demands of increased energy consumption. All this just in case! If our potential attacker proceeds to stick the knife in us, we bleed and a new set of reactions occur. These include going in to shock (where blood pressure falls dramatically, thus reducing potential blood loss), fainting and falling to the ground (thus aiding venous return), constriction of the veins (encouraging blood into the heart thereby forestalling heart failure) and a drop in temperature (which slows down our bodily functions). On top of all this, the process of clotting begins to seal up the wound.

If, on the other hand, the person with the knife walks straight past us to the place where a previously unseen birthday cake awaits, we sigh with relief and eventually start to relax. At this point, the parasympathetic nervous system takes over, heart rate and lung capacity decrease, the body ups the production of nitric oxide (which acts as an antidote to the stress hormones) and we begin the process of conserving and restoring energy, thus bringing the body back into a state of equilibrium.

What this example shows is that it is simply a physiological impossibility for us to be in a state of stress and a state of healing at the same time. The two states require the functioning of different bodily systems: either the *sympathetic* nervous system or the *parasympathetic* nervous system. Which we choose to activate depends on our state of mind. So, how ready are you to jump to negative conclusions? Are negative outcomes allowed to reaffirm your experiences more readily than positive ones? Does pessimism dictate your expectations? To what extent do you allow your emotional mindset to influence your physical wellbeing?

In our mainly affluent society, we are warm, fed and enjoy foreign holidays, leisure time, hobbies and pursuits undreamed of by previous generations. Yet, rather than feeling fulfilled, the tendency seems to be towards increased feelings of anxiety and ever-greater craving. The avaricious consumption of commodities that drives Western consumer societies will always fail to fill a hunger that stems from emotional emptiness. As long as we continue to seek answers outside of ourselves, in the guise of instant gratification or the acquisition of wealth and prestige, the mental dualism that this creates will continue to contribute towards the decline of our holistic health.

While the pressures of survival have changed subtly over the last one hundred years, humankind's psyche has yet to catch up. Life has always been a challenge but, for earlier generations, the traumas of infectious disease and resultant high infant mortality, famine and poverty were facts of life, beyond our control and therefore not our personal responsibility. Modern pressures, on the other hand, are very much pressures of self-responsibility. Are you good enough at your job? Did you fight hard enough for that promotion? Are you spending enough time with your children? Do you earn enough money to secure the future for yourself and your family? Indeed, a major industry is based on our most basic fear: what if the worst happens?' Rather than investing in our good health, we take out insurance on our expectation of bad health. This fear actually causes a stress response which then interferes with our body's natural inclination to be healthy. The result of these pressures is that, rather than succumbing to the killers of yesteryear, Western societies are manifesting a whole new range of diseases that result from internal imbalance and disharmony: cancer, heart disease, obesity, addiction and psychological breakdown.

The medical profession is very well aware that lifestyle leads to many forms of illness. They acknowledge, for example, that mental or emotional pressure can be an indicator of potential heart trouble, as the stress response is known to increase pressure on the heart. It has also been noted that cancer frequently shows up eighteen months to two years after the suffering of a particularly traumatic emotional event, such as bereavement, redundancy or divorce. But is this a result of the body's immune system being repressed during times of stress? Or is it that a subconscious message is sent to the self, confirming that there is no wish to go on in this life, either because of the desire to be reunited with the departed loved-one or because life without our usual support structure is simply no longer tolerable? Is it possible that at such times we send ourselves a literal self-destruct command and our ever-obedient bodies turn on themselves in the most effective way they know? It has been proven time and again that people who feel a strong sense of connection, who feel cared for and who have a strong and optimistic belief in their place in life will fare better than those who are isolated, fearful and lost. The act of reconnecting to ourselves and to our loved-ones finds its expression through the creation of a true home: a place that gives you the space to be yourself, that keeps the white noise of stress at bay and which nurtures happiness to the highest level possible. Only by ensuring that this, our emotional home, is in good order is it possible to embrace our true potential, which in turn will find its expression in physical health and harmony.

CHAPTER 11

❀ ❀ ˙ Making Sense of Design ❀ ❀

When thinking about designing the home, the tendency is to focus on aesthetic appearance. However, before we have even begun to intellectualize our responses to a given environment, we will have already responded on an intuitive level. To ensure that this intuitive reaction is a positive one, it is necessary to pay heed to the guiding principle behind the creation of a holistic home: comfort. For it is only by giving priority to our emotional and physical comfort that a house can ever truly succeed in becoming a home.

Originally, we built homes which instinctively respected our physical relationship to them: our size and our proportions dictated how much and what kind of space was needed. The out- stretched figure of man inclined early draftsmen towards the number five; so it was that the 5-sided pentagon and 5-pointed star-shape of the pentagram came to be recognized as a cornerstone of geometry and design. As humankind's awareness evolved, a set of principles was developed which was based more specifically on the proportional relationships mirrored between humankind and the cosmos. The system which these principles produced was called Sacred Geometry.

Sacred Geometry was considered by Plato to be key to the physics of harmony in the Universe, charting as it does the complex numerical journey that begins with a single Point, travels out to the Line, thence to the Second dimension (the plane), on to the Third (the solid) and beyond. It has been used in art and architecture ever since, but the cathedral at Chartres in France is perhaps its most beautiful embodiment. The calculations and realization of this wonderful building perfectly encapsulate the patterns and seeming coincidences at the heart of this universal understanding.

The founding mathematical relationship within Sacred Geometry is a ratio found repeatedly in nature and known as the Golden Section. Originally coined by Euclid over two-and-a-half thousand years ago, the Golden Section is arrived at by dividing a length in such a way that the ratio of the shorter part to the longer part is the same as the ratio of the longer part to the whole. This works out at roughly 1:1.68 or 8:13, simplified it translates as approximately 4:6. The home-maker can use this ratio to design anything from a set of cupboards to an entire room, as well as to hang pictures, mirrors, curtain tiebacks, dado rails and door handles at a height that works both instinctively and aesthetically. Le Corbusier, the Swiss architect of the previous century, claimed that the proportions of the ideal human being were embodied in the Golden Section and he developed a series of measurements based on a 6ft man to produce furniture and features sympathetic to the human form and spirit. These proportions are still in use today, now that ergonomic design is reasserting its relevance over the more idiosyncratic offerings of the last few decades.

Whilst Sacred Geometry informed humankind's earlier architectural accomplishments, in time our intuitive relationship with buildings was forgotten; instead, architecture came to be used symbolically: ever higher spires reaching to our God in Heaven, grander and grander buildings to reflect our increasing power and wealth and ever more complex security in order to protect us from the outside world. Today, many architects continue to ignore the intuitive interaction between people and their environment and so their structures succeed only as expressions of technical acumen and personal arrogance. As a result, these buildings are often difficult to remain in, causing subtle feelings of unease and even distress. However sophisticated humans and their technology become, it is still the case that the buildings which perform best in terms of their occupants' wellbeing are the ones that pay heed to the harmonious principles of Sacred Geometry.

When it comes to choosing a home, pay heed to this instinctive relationship and choose one that suits who you truly are, rather than who you think you should aspire to be. There is no point in trying to make money by buying a rambling wreck if the effort and stress involved in trying to do it up puts years on you. Nor will any good come from spending money on a large garden if gardening bores you and you can't afford a gardener. It will just be a source of stress. Whichever house you choose, make sure that it fits your family's size because there is a fine line between having adequate space for your needs and experiencing feelings of isolation or alienation within your own home. A home should resonate with life, with no room left un-warmed by daily use. During transitory times, such as before the arrival of anticipated offspring or later when they first leave home, try in their absence to create reasons for using all of the rooms, whether for hobbies, studies or exercise. The home is generally the biggest financial investment we make, so get the fundamentals right and you'll be on good foundations forever.

When deciding upon a style of decoration, allow the age and character of your building to be your guide in choosing sympathetic furnishings. Any property of any age can be successfully decorated provided that you remain true to the integrity of the building. A Victorian home will suit Victorian fittings far better than a modern semi-detached will. Similarly, a country cottage will always disappoint if you attempt to iron out its eccentricities with modern fixtures and fittings. Each of us has our own ideas about what is aesthetically pleasing and, as far as the holistic home is concerned, no one style is preferable to another. It's simply that one style may benefit a particular person and a particular house more than another may.

By thinking about what we want from our home, we can shape the way in which we interact with it. Do you love to lavish time and attention on it, or is it somewhere that has to look after you? Some styles are much easier to keep clean than others; if your days are busy or you find housework a chore, go for simple lines that don't attract dust and grease into difficult to clean nooks and crannies. For those with hectic schedules, the clean lines of a simple scheme can bring reprieve from the busyness of the day, allowing a calmness to descend on a mind distracted by decisions and deadlines. The trick to creating such a peaceful scheme is to limit the amount of contrasts within a room, whether these come from patterns, textures or objects. By choosing plain finishes and keeping the room uncluttered, the eye and brain are allowed a rest from information-overload. There is no need for such rooms to be minimalist in a cold or industrial sense. Hard surfaces such as chrome, stainless steel, glass and concrete may look fabulously stylish in a magazine but bring little comfort or respite. A tired body and exhausted spirit will be far better supported by an un-fussy but nevertheless welcoming mix of warm textures such as wood, cork, linoleum, sisal or wool, offset by the sumptuous richness of velvet, chenille and deep pile rugs.

Of course, very few people choose all their furnishings and decor at the same time. Most acquire a motley collection of inherited, donated, bought-when-it-could-be-afforded, hung-on-to for sentimental reasons, hung-on-to for reasons of laziness and "really must replace at some point" possessions, some of which are loved and some of which don't get looked at for years on end. In a therapeutic sense, it is our relationship to these possessions that is all-important so when assessing your home or embarking on any refurbishment, take the time to note your instinctive reaction to each particular item. Does it elicit a feeling of emotional comfort or discomfort? There is, for instance, no point lovingly redecorating the hall if you then re-hang the same picture that your partner loves but that you hate. Whatever the rest of the hall is doing, the picture will still be the first thing you see on entering your home and will still be subconsciously irritating you every time you see it. This is not the first emotion that your home should elicit! Similarly, that wonderful antique table that looks so beautiful by the front door will be less appealing if permanently covered with bills, keys and other of life's detritus. Again, not the first thing you want to see as you walk in the door or come down the stairs in the morning. Assessing your possessions in terms of their true value will allow you to see the rest for what it really is: clutter.

In the last few decades, clutter has become something of a public nuisance. Our love of spending has led to a glut of personal possessions, while the corporate love of new business means we are endlessly targeted with opportunities to acquire even more. In order to maintain stability in this sea of stuff, it is first necessary to separate clutter into two categories.

First there is the everyday type, things like bills, junk mail, the recycling or the never-mending pile, all of which can actually be dealt with very quickly and easily, bringing enormous satisfaction guaranteed. Unfortunately, the world in which we live conspires against us and, when we turn around, Bang! it's all come back again. Where you can, cut clutter off at source. Take the time to phone those mail order companies you bought one thing from ten years ago and request that you be deleted from their mailing list. Think about Direct Debit as a way of paying bills. Invest in an outside recycling station and make emptying it part of the weekly trip to the shops (or park or swimming pool). Sort through piles of mending and be honest about your skills. There are plenty of seamstresses out there who will happily repair that zip and bring your favourite skirt back into circulation within the week. Look at your list of 'Things To Do' and ask yourself what can easily be done. Many jobs are actually fairly minor but reap great benefits. Fixing up a towel rail may only require putting four screws in to the wall but it means no more wet towels hung over doors or left on the floor, getting pongy and never drying. Definitely time well invested. Take a fresh look around your home and note your reactions. How many jobs could and would be completed if you suddenly discovered that the in-laws or a film crew were descending in a week's time? Repair jobs rarely take up more energy than the energy we expend in putting them off, so if they can be done, do them.

The second type of clutter is rather more difficult to deal with as it tends to be made up of a lifetime's worth of memorabilia. The New Age counsellors advise us to de-clutter our lives, live in the moment and be free of attachment. These are all worthy aspirations but how many of us have actually evolved to that point? Only we, as individuals, can know what we are ready to let go of and what we still need to learn from. That is our journey, the reason we are here. To have someone else come into our lives and make judgements based on their own agenda is deeply harmful. Only get rid of items that have ceased to have meaning for you. If you have a box of childhood trinkets that you only take out to look at once every five years, no matter. Treasure them. As the years go by, some of the contents will no longer trigger memories for you and then you can let them go. Other possessions will move you still, sometimes to the extreme. These reactions show that there are still unresolved issues or feelings that are in some way stuck around this particular time, place or person. The item acts as a trigger for us to attend to these feelings and attempt to resolve them. Hopefully, this can be done and the associated pain floats away and the item is needed no more. Other items may move us to laughter and, whilst (hopefully) this reinforces our present happiness, it may act to remind us of the possibility of happiness, triggering a new appraisal of the present situation. What is important is that these memories are used to seek understanding and to release pain, fear or anger. If, on the other hand, these triggers are allowed to reinforce and further ingrain such feelings, we will never be free.

Listen to what your treasures are saying to you and resolve what you can.

Hopefully, most of the ornaments, photos, knick-knacks and artwork that surround us are reminders of happy times and loved-ones. But how often are these so-called treasures really looked at? Our brains are very adept at ignoring those things which they consider non-essential stimuli. This filtering system allows the brain to sift through the vast amount of sensory information that is fired at it, leaving it free to concentrate on anything that could affect our survival; after all, it's no good noticing the pretty flower but getting eaten by the tiger. This essential survival technique translates into a modern-day talent for ignoring ornaments and other non-threatening items. In order to keep some vibrancy in our homes, it is necessary to give meaning back to all those long-ignored trinkets, perhaps by sorting them into categories of those associated with summer and those with winter. These could then be rotated according to the seasons and the ceremony attached to the act of changeover will draw your eye and brain to them, bringing them alive. Furthermore, the space that appears between the now thinned-out ornaments acts to frame and highlight them. The added bonus is less dusting!

By ensuring that our houses contain only true treasures and are not simply overwhelmed by a lifetime's collection of clutter, vibrancy is maintained in our homes and our lives. This vibrancy allows energy to flow and true rest to manifest. A bedroom should be dedicated to relaxation (intimate or otherwise) and sleep. It should not double as an office, a dumping ground for clothes, bags or toys or a holding bay for the ironing. All these things serve to distract and so reawaken a mind that should be preparing for sleep. If you are short of space and the bedrooms have to be multi-purpose, invest in adequate storage so that these temptations and reminders of jobs to be done can be kept out of sight and remain out of mind. The apparent effort of tidying away is more concerned with habit than with actual work and the rewards of a good night's sleep amply repay the expenditure.

Emotional ease is as key to our enjoyment of a room as is the physical comfort afforded by any particular piece of furniture, so always take your habits into account when arranging your layout. Most small rooms have an inherent logic as far as furniture placement is concerned but it's the bigger rooms, especially a large sitting-room, that can leave us flailing around with the sheer possibility available. The temptation is often to emphasize the dimensions of the room by plastering the furniture around the sides and leaving a large space in the centre. What this space actually represents is a sort of communication vacuum: too wide for seated parties to communicate across without leaning forward and straining to hear and too fraught with the possibility of social mishap to be negotiated by any but the foolhardy. The other mistake is to place a low table in the centre of the space.

It will inevitably get filled up with junk (unless you are incredibly disciplined) and you will end up sitting around a kind of household compost heap. It is much better to split the room with subtle demarcations, such as a communal seating area occupying one part and a quieter reading corner with a comfy chair and it's own light source in another. Furniture can always be moved for that once-every-five-years gathering of more than six people; if it's generally just you, your partner and the dog then make the space cosy for the three of you.

A feature such as a fireplace will always give focus to a room and all but the most modern houses will have a chimney breast, if not a working fire. Originally, fireplaces formed the almost sacred heart of the home, with many cultures believing that this was the place where good or evil forces could enter the family fold. People would place talismans around the hearth to encourage benevolent energy in and to keep the malign at bay; this tradition survives to this day with many a mantle piece being home to precious objects and photos. Whether or not a fireplace is present, you can create a feeling of togetherness through the inclusive placement of furniture. Ensure that every seat in a given area is within the eye line of the others, thereby allowing for conversation without the twisting and straining of necks. Include a consolidating item, such as a circular rug or even a wall-hanging, and make sure that it contains the fiery colours of red, gold, orange or yellow to help gather together the energy of the family.

By thinking about our interaction with a given room, not only in terms of aesthetics but also on a physical and emotional level, a framework for design is created that truly enhances our holistic good health. The room will feel good to be in simply because our responses to it will be appropriate to the atmosphere and activity taking place within it. There will be no discordance: only harmony.

CHAPTER 12

❀ ❀ ❀   Colour Conscious   ❀ ❀ ❀

Colour is one of the most powerful components of our lives. Everything from heartbeat to mood is affected by the presence of colour in the form of light energy. In terms of interior design, it is the biggest single design statement that you can make and, as such, will have a major impact on how you experience both your home and your health.

Colour has the power to elicit very real physical and emotional responses, both universally (as experienced by each and every one of us) and also personally, dependent on any particular associations we may have with it as individuals. But with such a vast range of colours and finishes available, one can become blinded by the sheer possibility on offer and so lose touch with our intuitive response to any given tint or shade. Yet it is only by acknowledging these responses and designing accordingly that schemes can be created which support the user both in themselves and in the activity for which the room is intended. Rooms that are colour conscious do more than just aesthetically please: they become active therapy.

From the moment we open our eyes we are subject to the pervasive effects of colour. The pure white light of the Sun flows in a wide electromagnetic spectrum that radiates in both visible and invisible wave forms. On hitting the retina in the eye, signals are transmitted to the brain via the optic nerve, allowing light activated information to be sent out around the body via the actions of the hormonal system. Colour appears as these electromagnetic waves have different lengths and vibratory speeds. The colours at the blue and violet end of the spectrum have shorter wavelengths and faster vibratory rates and appear to the eye to recede. This means that the brain interprets them as being non-threatening and they therefore act to calm and soothe us. Yellow, orange and red have longer, slower wavelengths and as they appear to advance towards us, act to warm and stimulate our physical responses. Green at the centre reflects perfect balance and as such is the colour associated with health and growth.

The primary colours of light are red, green and blue-violet, which when blended give white light. (As opposed to the primary colours of pigment which are red, blue and yellow and combine to make black.) Our perception of colour occurs as any given surface either absorbs or reflects particular light rays. A green apple absorbs all the colour rays except green and so that is what is seen. If this green apple were to be placed under a red light it would appear black, as the fruit absorbs the red light. It is this filtering system that allows some colour energy in and keeps others out. Consequently, a person who is habitually surrounded by one particular colour, eats only limited foods or remains in bland environments will begin to experience the distorting affects of colour imbalance. Each vibration has a specific physiological impact on us, but whilst science has only recently begun making use of invisible wavelengths, in radios, microwaves, x-rays and television, nature has been making use of colour for a millennia. In the natural world, colour is used to show off or to camouflage, to give warning or to attract. The delicate Bee Orchid has created a convincing representation of a bee in its petal colours and uses this arrangement to attract a real bee to the sweet nectar hidden within its flower. In a similar way, the colours found in fruit and vegetables alert us to the fact that they are high in particular nutrients. Green vegetables such as broccoli, cabbage and Brussels sprouts tend to be high in cancer-busting properties such as indoles and dithiolthiones, whilst carrots, peppers and sweet potatoes share not only similar hues of red/orange but also a similarly high percentage of beta-carotenes. When vegetables are over-cooked, colour leaches out of them and nutrients are lost, indicating that the relationship between plants and nutrition goes beyond just vitamins and minerals to include the presence of some kind of therapeutic colour energy.

Colour power has been harnessed for therapeutic benefit for centuries. In the first century A.D., the scholar Pliny wrote of the use of green lenses made from *smaragdus* (emeralds or other greenish minerals) to provide a soothing effect on tired eyes. He reported that, after straining to look at another object, the eyesight could be restored to normal by looking at a *smaragdus*. This fact was particularly appreciated by engravers of gemstones, who found this to be the most agreeable means of refreshing their eyes.

Later, in the 19th century, the revolutionary thinker Edwin Babbit put forward his theory that all humans, animals and plants were composed of components that had specific colour associations. In 1878, his book, *The Principles of Light and Colour*, detailed studies which showed how various ailments could be positively affected by exposure to certain coloured light. During the 1950s, the publication of Faber Birren's book, *Colour Psychology and Colour Therapy*, brought the physiological and psychological impact of colour to a new generation of design professionals and manufacturers, who in turn used this knowledge to create user-orientated environments and packaging. In the field of science, physics took humankind's understanding further with the revelation that all things in the universe are made up of energy packets. Entities, including ourselves, are not in fact solid but are made up of vibrating particles of energy which are then organized into interacting fields of force. This concurs with the belief held by many that our physical bodies are the densest manifestation of our personal energy-field and that each individual also has lighter energetic bodies, the densities of which are indicated by colours visible only to the attuned eye.

Awareness of the presence of these light bodies and energy-fields has been referred to many times throughout our history. In the 12th century, scholars Boirac and Liebeault noted the non-verbal, non-sight-led inter-action that occurred between humans even at a distance and recognized that this implied communication pathways and levels of interaction beyond the physical plane. However, it was not until the development of corona dis-charge photography, pioneered by Semyon Kirlian in the 1950s, that the presence of these personal energy-fields was confirmed and their composi-tion analysed objectively.

The chakras are energetic centres occurring at specific points along the body. When these centres are open, they allow energetic nourishment to flow into the personal field (or aura) of the individual. Throughout history, the perception of this colour energy has often been interpreted as a divine (rather than an energetic) manifestation; classical paintings of Christ fre-quently show golden rays radiating from his body, or his heart painted green, the colour associated with the heart chakra.

The main chakras correspond to the seven major nerve plexuses of the physical body, with each appearing to the sensitive eye as a different colour representing a different energy. When these chakras are closed, energy is blocked from reaching us, causing us to become deficient, weakened and ill. A healthy body should be awash with the colours of this light energy but if colours are dulled or absent a deficiency is indicated, implying depleted resources and imbalance. It is possible to attract any particular colour energy that may be lacking simply by introducing that colour back into our lives through the food we eat, the décor surrounding us, the clothes we wear and the plants, jewellery (particularly crystals) and objects we have around us.

What follows is a chart showing how colour energy affects our physical and emotional beings via the chakra points of the body.

See if you recognize any correlation with your own experience.

Chakra	Associated colour	Physical/emotional influence
Crown	White/Violet	Upper brain; pineal gland; anti-inflammatory; spiritually calming.
Brow	Indigo	Nervous system; pituitary gland; the physical senses; inspiration; intuition.
Throat	Blue	Vocal and bronchial tract; thyroid gland; respiratory system; physical and spiritual communication; anti-inflammatory.
Heart	Green	Heart; thymus gland; circulatory system; blood; emotionally and physically harmonizing; flow of love.
Solar plexus	Yellow	Stomach; liver; gall bladder; pancreas; nervous and hormonal strength; mental and emotional balance; wisdom.
Navel	Orange	Sexual organs; reproductive system; mental, physical and spiritual pleasure; shock absorber; cleansing and revitalizing of physical/etheric body.
Base	Red	Adrenal glands; muscular system; kidneys; physicality; reality; spiritual grounding.

Whether our relationship with colour is an emotional association or a universal physical response can be difficult to define. For example, although red causes a rise in blood pressure, is this because of the particular physical effect of that frequency wave-length or simply that, for our whole evolution, red has been associated with either blood or fire, both of which elicit a stress response? Is the colour green associated with growth because of its association with living plants, or because consuming those plants causes a healthy response from our own living tissue?

Some effects of colour are more obviously associative as there are distinct cultural differences. In European cultures, black is associated with death: in India, white is the colour associated with mourning. Religions also create associations; for example, orange denotes humility for Buddhists, but to western eyes it is a colour of flamboyance.

With this in mind, look at the colours with which you surround yourself. Your present choices are a subconscious message, what are they saying to you? Is there one colour to which you are particularly drawn? Is there one that you avoid? Think hard about the time when this colour was last in your life. What was happening at that time?

The following chart shows the emotional qualities associated with each colour, as well as the problems that can manifest if there is too little or too much of each. Remember: there are no good or bad colours, only imbalance.

Colour / energy	too little	too much
Red/energy, passion, life-force.	Lethargy, inactivity, insipidity.	Aggression, being hyped-up, inflammation.
Orange/joy, creativity, expression.	Depression, mundanity, boredom.	Over-excitability, taxing.
Yellow/mental alacrity, optimism, intellectual clarity.	Pessimism, insularity, narrow-mindedness.	Being physically and emotionally overwrought, egocentricity, irrationality.
Green / balance, harmony, healing.	Disengagement from self and from world around.	Procrastination, inability to move on.
Blue / contemplation, calm, relief.	Lack of vision, inability to breathe in life.	Depression, withdrawal from physical reality.
Purple / truth, justice, spirituality.	Lack of inspiration and faith, hopelessness.	Judgement, high-handed-ness, imbalance.
White / purity, cleanliness.	Being cluttered and muddled.	Isolation, being uncon-nected.
Brown / grounding, earthy.	Being ungrounded, rest-lessness, twitchiness.	Being in a rut or bogged down.
Pink / love: given and received freely.	Lack of sureness, needi-ness, lack of care for self.	Immaturity, lack of confidence, clinginess.
Turquoise / refreshing, effervescent, brilliant.	Loss of vitalizing energy.	Coolness, being unknow-able.
Grey / serenity, being at peace, self-containment	Fear of the void, attitude of grasping.	Detachment, lack of caring, aloofness.

Being aware of the impact of colour is particularly important when creating rooms for the more vulnerable members of the family, such as the very young, the very old or the poorly. For matters of chronic or acute ill-health, the help of a colour therapist is recommended; otherwise, remember that the keywords are balance and harmony. For those who are frail or vulnerable, choose a soft, lighter saturation of tone in order not to overwhelm a sensitive soul. A newborn baby, having only recently left the physical and energetic protection of the womb, will be engulfed by a whole new field of influence. As the process of their awakening to the physical world continues, their sensitivity is such that the parent must do all they can to soften the energy around them. The anger of an adult seems like a tornado to a baby and so, too, will loud music and bright primary colours. Only by using the subtlest tones, vocally and visually, do you allow your baby to gently assimilate the newness of their world. Furthermore, it is important to ensure full spectrum development by allowing access to a full representation of *all* the colour energies; disregard the whole blue for boys / pink for girls nonsense.

Stronger saturations of colour can safely be introduced as the child grows and their sense of self strengthens. Their bedroom is the ideal place for them to explore and develop their creativity; the more respect afforded to them in this the better. Allowing a child to decorate their own room, especially on arrival in a new house, gives them the opportunity to establish themselves in their new environment and gives vent to any emotional needs or creative impulses. Yellow is associated with developing mental acumen, whilst red is the embodiment of all that is physical. A love of bright colours shows a happy, confident child. A liking for black does not mean that they are into devil worship (though the presence of skulls may be a clue!), only that they feel the need to create a kind of protective cloak around themselves whilst they work out their place in the scheme of things. As a phase, black offers the chance for reflection and meditation, the space in which to explore feelings and emotions. In China, black is associated with the feminine energy of the universe and as a child reaches adulthood, the need for the protective, maternal warmth of the womb is symbolized by being drawn towards the deep, encompassing tones of black. If black remains dominant for too long, however, the effect becomes oppressive and stifling. The pattern becomes a habit and inhibits the person's expression of their true worth. Again, this demonstrates how overexposure to any particular colour can cause problems.

The more settled periods of adulthood can often result in our establishing and ingraining colour habits; those safe and familiar hues which bring comfort but little in the way of inspiration or balance. Those who stick doggedly to one colour may be afraid of experimentation or simply lack the energy for change, but the gentle introduction of new colours (even as fleeting as a bunch of flowers) can begin to open the channel that will eventually allow a person to move forward. Occasionally, having spent years favouring a particular hue, one may find oneself being drawn to an altogether different colour. This indicates that a period of transition is beginning, opening the door to new directions.

With the onset of old age, many are attracted to the mauves and lilacs which connect us to the celestial plane and which are symbolic of the wisdom associated with a long life. Finally, as death approaches, the colour seems to float away from our hair, our skin and our eyes. Often, it is only then that those who look on become aware of the true colour of this, our life force.

When choosing colours for our home, we not only send a message about ourselves but we also have a physiological and emotional impact on those with whom we share our home. The stay-at-home partner may love the colour yellow; it is, after all, the most popular colour in decoration amongst adults today. Unfortunately, the out-to-work partner may well have faced endless exposure to yellow lighting in offices, train carriages, from street lights and car headlights. Coming home to the *feng shui*-ed yellow of the front door, the sunny primrose yellow of the kitchen and the golden warmth of the sitting room, all lit by yet more yellow-biased lighting, will stimulate the brainwaves beyond that which is healthy. While a little yellow is good at making one alert and clear-headed, too much leaves us mentally-hyped, without anchorage or grounding. An excess of yellow encourages nervousness and irritability, eventually causing a susceptible individual to become egocentric and fearful. This paranoia may lead to arguments and even violence. Sounds familiar? Change the paintwork and notice the difference.

As you begin to decorate, consider the dominating atmosphere in your home as it is at the moment: is it harmonious or is there discord? Do you tend to gravitate towards each other or does everyone disappear in to their own space as quickly as possible? Are you interested in each other's day or tetchy as a result of your own? Look back at the chart denoting the effects that each of the colour energies brings. Is there a correlation? Use these answers as well as the input of your family to create rooms that work for everyone. If everyone feels a part of the creative process, they are more likely to remain engaged once the decorating is complete. Bearing in mind, then, that each of us has our own colour needs and prejudices, let's now look at some suggestions for each room, always remembering some basic rules of thumb.

Firstly, balance. Try to ensure that all colours are represented throughout the house as a whole and that no one colour dominates.

Secondly, for rooms that are to be used socially, the primary need is to feel warm; it therefore makes sense to use colours from the warming end of the spectrum i.e. red, orange and yellow. On the other hand, when our bodily systems (circulatory, respiratory, nervous and so on) need to relax, it is the cooling tones of blue, green and purple which tend to benefit us.

When creating a scheme for a large family group, a neutral background allows you to represent all other colour energies through cushion-covers, rugs, artwork, plants and other accessories. A neutral base scheme also works for those in a period of transition or for any who may be presently unsure of how to progress, as it allows new colours to be introduced as and when you feel drawn to them. For anyone feeling emotionally vulnerable, it is helpful to gain inspiration from the colours found in nature as their energies symbolize the grounding and growth necessary for healing.

If you are beginning a room from scratch, always start by choosing your textiles first. It's much easier to match paint to fabric than vice versa. For a foolproof method of achieving a perfectly co-ordinated and beautifully balanced scheme, begin by choosing your patterned fabric. Then match your wall paint to the background colour of the fabric and your accessories to the stronger colours highlighted in the pattern. By matching your wall paint to the palest colour present, you will bring a calm, fresh feel to your scheme. Alternatively, you could match it with the deepest shade for heightened drama.

Using a token representation of a complementary colour, i.e. one that comes from the opposite side of the colour wheel, will energize the main colour and bring the room alive. To find the exact complement to any particular hue, simply find a large blank sheet of plain white paper and place a circle of your chosen colour on the left-hand side of the sheet. Allow your eyes to 'drink' in this colour for a minute or so and then look immediately at the blank area of the paper on the right. Before your eyes will manifest the exact complementary colour to the colour upon which you've just been focusing. Combining these colours as light would create white light which contains the full spectrum, thereby bringing the balance which the body craves. However, make sure that you use no more than 10% of the complementary colour to the main. Equal or similar amounts of the two colours will be draining, as their energies effectively fight for your attention, leaving the atmosphere hanging literally in the balance. Split complementaries also work well. This is where you use a main colour, such as soft yellow (cream) with the highlights of the complementary violet split into lavender (a warm blue) and heather (a cool red).

When using warm and cool-toned colours together, it is more successful to use pale, warm colours and deep, cool colours than vice versa. Think of soft orange and deep blue as opposed to deep orange and pale blue or purple and primrose as opposed to lavender and gold.

When choosing a wall colour, think of what will be reflected on to it. Lots of sunlight with pale cupboards and flooring will give a different end-result than will dark surfaces and a north-facing window. As a general principle, go slightly lighter than your initial choice; in most rooms, the walls will reflect back on themselves, making the finished effect look darker.

Intense colours reflect less light and so tend to make a room look darker and smaller, but do not let this put you off using rich, jewel-like hues in a small room. They will take on a life and definition of their own that makes size immaterial.

The sitting room is usually the most communal room in the house; for that reason, a scheme should be chosen that is warm and comforting without being overpowering. As a general rule, use soft, earthier tones of warm colours (such as burnt orange or yellow ochre) that will not jar at the end of a long day. If, however, your family is very argumentative, steer clear of strong yellows (which can stimulate the brain into paranoid overdrive) and pure reds (with their associated heightened physicality). Orange brings together the earthy energy of red and the intellectual energy of yellow, the effect of the combination being to rationalize the physicality of red whilst grounding the mental flow of yellow. If there is actual violence, whether verbal or physical, steer clear of these stimulating colours altogether and go for warm browns and soft pinks which have been successfully used both in prisons and secure mental institutions to calm violent inmates. The power of colour is not to be under-estimated.

Warm colours are also recommended for the kitchen but, again, take into account the needs of the primary cook. Soft, grounding tones will inspire a tired body without overly-stimulating a mind exhausted after a long working day.

Occasionally, the preparation and consumption of food becomes a more complex issue and whether this is because of ill-health, negative associations or emotional needs colour can be used to support rather than excite. The calming tones of lavender, plum or aubergine will create a soothing, reassuring scheme that encourages and supports sensitive eaters without appearing challenging or overwhelming. Alternatively, use the freshness of green to enhance our connection with nature and bring a lightness to both the room and to patterns of cooking and eating.

Dining rooms tend to be used less often than the other rooms and, for this reason, often occupy the north-facing side of the house. However, it is not healthy to have certain rooms unused within the home as they will soon feel stagnant; if you wish to get more use from your dining room, choose the colours of gold, red or orange to invite energy in. If your dining room is sunny and frequently-used and you wish to use blues or greens as a colour scheme, use tones of midnight blue and deep sea-green which simply melt away when the candles are lit. With the colours of fire as your table-setting, you can re-create the feel of the campfire under the eternal sky, encouraging the instinct to gather round and share stories and intimacies as in the days of old. Remember that your dinner party will be far livelier if everyone is feeling hearty, animated and connected to one another.

After the excitement and possible trials of the day, what's needed is a relaxing bath and a restorative night's sleep. After the bright lights of the office, the journey home and the television, think of balance once again and it will guide you to the cooler colours of green, blue and purple. Pink can also be used successfully in a bathroom or bedroom, as it acts as a muscle-relaxant, but be aware of its propensity towards girlishness and always use an earthy rather than a zingy tone.

As soon as these colours hit the retina, the process of relaxing begins. What should be borne in mind, however, is that the desired effect is to *calm* down not *chill* down and, whilst a bedroom has the warmth of multi-layered soft furnishings to take the edge off cool hues, bathrooms are a different proposition and require more care. Here, the effect of a cool blue or green is hardened by the presence of unforgiving surfaces such as tiles, porcelain, marble, cement, plastic and pipes.

Strong, vivid tones such as tropical turquoise or Mediterranean blue precisely suit those climates, with their bright sunshine and intense heat, but become rather stark and slightly overpowering in cooler, northern climes. Such rooms make us feel cold and our mirrored reflections look drained and ill, not at all conducive to feeling restored. If you wish to use blue or green, pick a tone that has been warmed and softened by a slightly yellow, red or greyish undertone, such as eau de nil, lavender, duck egg blue or sage. If your bathroom is in any way cold or uninviting, it is better instead to create a softer scheme using the other colours associated with the sea: the rich colours of coral, the pinks and yellows of sand or the pretty opalescence of shell.

Many people now work from home and, even for those who do not, the computer is becoming an increasingly essential household appliance. Whether for work or leisure, the colour chosen for the backdrop is all-important. The brain perceives greens, blues and purples as being non-threatening and therefore safe to ignore, which helps to minimize the eye-strain caused by the computerized words and images. In a cool dark room, warmer tones of these receding colours (such as lavender, petrol blue or celadon green) are best whereas in a hot, bright room something cooling and minty can be effective. It is very easy to physically chill down when working at a computer, so bear this propensity to coolness in mind when choosing colours for an office space.

As you can see, colour choices are both revealing and inspiring. The writing really is on the wall, so make sure that the colour message you send to yourself is one that heals.

Light As Therapy

Humankind has long recognized that the sunlight which bathes our planet is a fundamental prerequisite to life on Earth. Up until the 1960s, heliotherapy was a respected means of exploiting the benefits of this natural energy source, being used to treat illnesses such as tuberculosis, smallpox and wounds. Regular exposure to natural, full spectrum daylight allows for the maintenance of healthy human functioning, including the regulation of body temperature, hormonal balance, tissue growth, restorative sleep and mental alertness. All are dependent on the body's being in tune with the passage of our planet around the Sun. However, it is only now that the many ways in which the body utilizes this life-giving energy: electrical, chemical, osmotic and mechanical is being fully understood.

The ultraviolet rays found in full spectrum sunlight act to stimulate a form of cholesterol found in the oil of the skin, converting it to a form of vitamin D. This vitamin is crucial in facilitating the body's absorption of calcium and phosphorus, as well as for the formation of strong bones and teeth. Sunlight is also absorbed through the eyes, stimulating the pituitary and pineal glands situated in the brain. The function of these glands includes the storage and release of the hormones responsible for thyroid and adrenal function, as well as for growth, fluid balance and regulation of the reproductive organs. Hormones are inextricably linked to our emotions and any imbalance can cause a wide range of psycho-physiological manifestations. Most of us have, at some point, experienced disruption to the established pattern of our days and nights such as a long haul flight, caring for a newborn or doing shift work. The fatigue and malaise induced by interrupted sleep and wakefulness patterns is an indicator of just how dependent our wellbeing is on the circadian rhythm of the natural day. The official recognition of Seasonal Affective Disorder (SAD) has brought relief to thousands of people who suffer every year as the days shorten and the hours of sunlight decrease. Now that the association has been made between the emotional symptoms of depression, lethargy and social withdrawal and the physical lowering of melatonin levels secreted by the pineal gland during winter, this debilitating condition can be simply and effectively alleviated by daily exposure to bright light. Ensuring a daily walk of at least 30 minutes in the fresh air will help maintain not only your cardiovascular health but also your hormonal, skeletal, nervous and immune systems as well.

At school, children are taught that plants use the process of photosynthesis to absorb light energy via their green-pigmented chlorophyll and that it is this light which allows them to flourish. However, the molecular processes employed by the human body have always been harder to assess. For, although a vegetable-rich diet has long been recognized as necessary for good health, our appreciation has been limited to its vitamin and mineral content. Now, however, scientists working in the field of biophysics are starting to discover a far more dynamic relationship between food and health; what their work shows is that light energy is playing a significant role not only in the health of the plant, but in the health of those who then eat it.

Biophysics suggests that the body utilizes light in the form of photons to receive, organize and emit the energy necessary for healthy functioning. Organisms are seen to actively seek out this essential energy source whether they are flowers turning their faces to the Sun or humans flocking outdoors on the first bright days of spring. Fritz-Albert Popp, a biophysicist working at the University of Marberg, developed a machine capable of counting light, photon by photon; he suggests that this gulping of light (or 'photon-sucking' as he terms it) excites the electrons in the body, literally winding it up for action. He concludes that a lack of regular access to this vibrational life energy causes the organism to become literally run-down, as the once-stimulated electrons slowly but inevitably grind to a halt. Further studies by Popp suggest that, in a state of perfect health, photons are organized in a coherent, rhythmical pattern. Ill-health, on the other hand, causes either a fatal repression of this light or an overwhelming surge of it. What his work demonstrates is that light forms the communication pathway by which an organism (even one as complex as ourselves) organizes not only its own growth and development but also its continuing inner equilibrium and health. Full spectrum sunlight, accessed by the consumption of nutritionally-vibrant food and time spent in the natural world, is used by the body to repair damaged cells and maintain health on a molecular level. When denied sunlight, this photo-repair mechanism is prevented, resulting in the cells' natural intelligence becoming scrambled, the result being imbalance and disease.

As light therapy comes once again into the spotlight, it is returning to the forefront of healing technology. Its potential for treating viruses (including those associated with AIDS) is being explored by scientists in the U.S. while, in the U.K., photodynamic therapy is using light to enhance the effect of chemotherapy drugs in the destruction of malign tumours.

Unfortunately, between our unpredictable climate and urbanized lifestyle, it seems that we are spending more time indoors than is healthy for us. Whatever the weather, strive to ensure that part of each day is spent in untinted, unshaded natural daylight and, for the time that has to be spent indoors, do all that you can to make full use of the light available.

First of all, pay attention to the orientation of your home. Before allocating rooms in a new house, take the time to follow the path of the Sun and get in touch with the natural cycles that govern our lives. If you have trouble waking up in the morning, it makes sense to situate the bedroom in an east-facing room in order to access the energy and light of the rising Sun. On the other hand, if you want to sleep on in the mornings, a west-facing room will allow for prolonged shut-eye. Activity rooms (such as kitchen, play- and living-rooms) should be given priority access to any available sunlight, whereas rooms that are used less often can cope with being on the north-facing side of the house. Mirrors can be placed on walls opposite the window to reflect extra daylight into any rooms that are naturally lacking in light.

Ensure that you make the most of what natural light there is. Keep the sills clear and, if the window overlooks a garden, keep the shrubs immediately outside the window trimmed back. Make sure that windows are cleaned regularly, especially in polluted inner-cities and try not to block incoming light with overly-elaborate drapes. If possible, extend curtain poles beyond the window width to allow the drawn-back curtains to frame the window rather than obscure it. Using tie-backs will ensure that as much light as possible enters the room. Venetian blinds, or the softer Roman version, can be pulled up to leave a minimal impact on window space, while sheer fabrics can be used to gently filter natural light, so helping to protect delicate furnishings or give privacy without blocking the daylight out completely. There are some beautiful colours and patterns on the market, but remember that these will fade in the summer in a matter of weeks; unless you choose white, they should be used in conjunction with a blind and tied out of the direct rays of the Sun. Using two forms of window dressing like this allows light to be manipulated as required. For example, a heavier material can be in place to ensure evening privacy, then drawn back to leave only a sheer covering to the first rays of the morning Sun. This can be a real asset to those who find getting up in the mornings a struggle. Alternatively, many people (particularly young children or those who feel emotionally vulnerable) feel uncomfortable in pitch darkness and find the soft light of the Moon or street-lights soothing. In the case of young children, a little parental intervention once they are asleep can close the heavier curtain or blind in order to prevent early waking.

Ensuring optimal access to daylight is fundamental in designing a health-conscious home but artificial light can be used to augment what is naturally available, create interest and add a further dimension to an interior scheme. Most home lighting tends to come from incandescent bulbs which give off a red light that tinges everything yellow. It is important to bear this in mind when choosing colours for walls, as an incandescent bulb will turn a white wall cream and a pink wall brown. This can result in your carefully chosen wall lights creating pools of muddiness on the very walls they were meant to enhance. Remember, also, that incandescent bulbs give off a lot of infrared heat, causing a build-up if they are used for spot- or directional-lighting. This is obviously undesirable, so ensure that any spotlights that are aimed at work surfaces don't in fact hit you on the back of your head; not only will you be casting a shadow on to your workspace but you will get a headache as well.

The other type of frequently-used bulb is the standard fluorescent. These give off a blue or ultraviolet light which can cause eyestrain and make one feel cold and somewhat below par. Studies indicate that standard fluorescent lighting produces a significantly higher reaction from the stress hormones than does full spectrum lighting. When these lights age, they can give off a barely-noticeable flicker that is at odds with our own natural vibratory rate. Because of this they are often implicated in making people feel irritable, hyperactive or even in inducing fits. If you feel prone to this type of complaint, change any fluorescent bulbs immediately. Often, offices and shops use this form of lighting as the newer models are more energy-efficient, but if you are finding that your eyes are becoming sore or that you are experiencing any other symptoms potentially attributable to this, make sure that your bosses know about it and take action.

The best form of lighting is tungsten-halogen lights. They are close in quality to daylight and the low voltage ones are extremely energy-efficient. The initial cost may seem expensive, but their long life means that they will save you money in the end. If your work requires any kind of precision, whether of technique or colour purity, then top-quality lighting is a prerequisite and investing in this form of lighting will definitely pay dividends.

Coloured light can be used therapeutically in the same way as coloured pigment. Pink light is therefore relaxing and nurturing, orange joyful and stimulating, red warming and exciting. At the more soothing end of the spectrum, green light is found to be both healing and calming and so is recommended for relaxing and recuperating after illness. Blue light will help cool a fever or soothe a hyperactive child while both blue and ultra-violet light have been used to treat conditions such as psoriasis and herpes simplex and, in particular, neo-natal jaundice. (Note that yellow jaundice and the blue/mauve of the light come from opposite sides of the colour wheel, thereby creating balance.) Full spectrum lights are available which represent the full balance found in sunlight. However, ultra-violet light is recommended for therapeutic uses only, as it can raise levels beyond that which is regarded as generally safe, especially when used in a room that contains electrical equipment. Because of these concerns, full spectrum lights are now available which omit this particular ray; these have also been shown to improve both performance and mood. Any light with a soothing colour bias will leave one feeling quite sleepy and enervated so they are not recommended for use when undertaking even light mental tasks, such as watching television, as they will cause eye-strain and tiredness. Any coloured light should be used carefully with full regard to its therapeutic qualities.

Having become aware of the implications of the colour inherent in lighting, think about the atmosphere that you are attempting to create. Do you need soft, ambient lighting created by wall-washers and low-level lamps, or is it a work room requiring directional lighting provided by spotlights and angle-poises? Do you require an overall brightness provided by recessed fittings or a central feature, such as a chandelier, over a dining table? Remember that in the office or the sitting-room, you need to ensure that there are no lights reflected in your computer or television screen. Any that do reflect will increase eye-strain and susceptibility to tiredness. If your office space has overhead fluorescent lighting (as many do), try to ensure that your screen sits at right angles to it, so diminishing the amount of reflection.

These days there are many wonderful and whimsical lighting options available. Fairy lights now frequently show their colourful display all year round and strings of single-coloured lighting are used to highlight everything from picture rails to artwork to indoor trees. Chinese lanterns and rose-bower styles bring a taste of something more exotic to both inside and out, whilst light panels and boxes give a cutting edge to the art of illumination. The many forms of lighting now available are both playful and creative; remember, though, that most are not necessarily practical as far as actually shedding light is concerned.

The final consideration is the size of the room which you are illuminating. An 8-pronged chandelier, complete with 60watt bulbs, will overwhelm a 12-foot square room and give everyone a headache. The aim is to be as flexible as possible, especially in rooms that are used for a variety of purposes; by combining the fanciful with the functional, maximum versatility is created. Dimmer switches are not recommended as they simply create an overall murkiness; it is better instead to create pools of illumination that allow an interplay of light and shadow. Teaming lamps and wall lights with a wall-covering that has a soft sheen elicits a glow reminiscent of candlelight, thus bringing a richness and warmth to any room.

The most important thing to remember is that we are all spending more time under artificial light than is healthy either for ourselves or the planet. Use appropriate levels of lighting to prevent eye-strain but, beyond that, less is most definitely more.

❀ ❀ ❀   The Sensual Home   ❀ ❀ ❀

It is our senses that allow us to experience the world; what we see, hear, smell, touch and taste guides us through the physical landscape and provides us with the reference bank of information required to negotiate new challenges.

Having received this sensory information, the brain then responds on both a conscious and a subconscious level. For instance, when we register intense heat on our fingertips we instantaneously withdraw them from the source of that heat. We may then consciously choose to put our fingers in our mouth to reduce the heat, pain and chance of infection, whilst *sub*consciously a blister is formed to protect the vulnerable area and to promote healing. The experience and our reactions to it affirm our wariness of hot items and our future ability to respond effectively to them.

As new-born babies develop, they come to embody their experiences and to reflect them back, beginning the process that ultimately creates their own sense of reality. Within a very few weeks, a baby begins to associate the receiving of smiles with happy, comfortable situations and shortly after that comes the realization that the proffering of smiles can influence situations for the better. A child who experiences the security of a happy, harmonious home will reflect that in their disposition and therefore be more likely to encounter positive reactions from others. The frequency and type of sensory experiences encountered from this early age form our worldview; it is this worldview that is then reflected back out into the collective arena. With the arrival of adulthood, those early experiences can be reinforced or, if necessary, new and more positive ones can be created.

If all senses are lost through reasons of ill-health or injury, a sensory void known as deep coma is entered. However, when only one or two senses are lost, such as sight or hearing, the remaining senses will often sharpen while, sometimes, the previously ignored sixth sense of psychic ability develops. This may well come as a result of losing some of the white noise that so interferes with our day-to-day experience; after all, it is difficult to hear the small quiet voice of intuition if the clanging sound of advertising is ringing in our ears. Neither can one expect to perceive auras if the eyes are straining to see the television, the Internet and the latest gossip column.

Although it is the visual and aural senses that seem to be the most targeted by daily events, our other senses are also crucial to our burgeoning understanding of the world and the events around us. Smell, for example, activates the very deep part of our brain associated with storing memories, meaning that experiencing certain smells can transport us back to a time that predates even our earliest visual recollections.

When creating a holistically comfortable home, one must pay attention to all of the senses and avoid overloading any one in particular. The brain is besieged by a sensory onslaught every moment of every day; even in sleep it is still alert to the vibrations of the world around it. It works very hard at processing these vast amounts of information into what it needs to recognize for survival and what it can safely ignore. This filtering effect should always be borne in mind because, as was discussed earlier, anything that is fixed be it an ornament, a smell or a sound ceases to be noticed by the brain and instead becomes simply clutter.

With this in mind, what do your senses tell you as you enter your home? At this point it's often good to ask a friend for their immediate impressions, as they will be much more objective about your home than you will. For instance, they may notice a certain doggy smell without necessarily associating it with that adorable creature in the basket. Alternatively, they may experience a slight awkwardness as they shuffle through the partially-opened door, past the pile of coats and down a long, brightly-lit corridor to the reception room. They've been in your home for several minutes before they are allowed to exhale properly. These first impressions can give form to how our home is experienced by all who enter and that includes the household, even though they may have stopped consciously noting their reactions. In this way, our homes (and therefore ourselves) will always be re-revealing themselves to newcomers but, by increasing our overall awareness, a degree of clarity and peacefulness can be consciously manifested that will make the home a more pleasingly sensuous experience.

As previous chapters have already discussed the visual impact of style, colour and light, this chapter will focus on the more subtle realms of touch, scent and sound. The sensation of taste is yet another information channel, although much of what we think of as taste is, in fact, smell.

TOUCH

Our sense of touch is our earliest reliable source of information. Long before we learn to recognize objects by sight, we use our hands and mouths to determine their nature. Are they yielding or hard? Are they warm or cold? Can I grasp it or will doing so cause me pain? As we grow older and our experience and memory-bank builds, we come to rely less heavily on touch as an information channel, yet these early tactile experiences are vital in establishing our world as being either safe and comfortable or inconsistent and dangerous.

Within the home, our sense of touch is accommodated by the variety of textures that are chosen to cover walls, floors, furniture and furnishings. By becoming aware of the inherent feel of a surface, rather than simply focusing on its look, an environment can be created that refreshes, embraces, grounds or inspires, as appropriate to the needs of each room and its occupants. Unfortunately, a lot of modern furniture design is concerned with aesthetics rather than experience. The smart interiors featured in magazines can look stylish but, at the same time, leave you feeling cold, the reason being that you would actually begin to feel physically chilled as your muscles tense against the inherent discomfort and cool tones of these design masterpieces. One such example is the trend for designing private kitchens to look like commercial ones, complete with stainless steel units and strong lighting. The reason why commercial kitchens opt for this design is that they are essentially meal factories; they are where the creativity of the chef is realized and are therefore more about supply than inspiration. Once in the home, the practical qualities of stainless steel and bright light translate into a cold, clinical environment where creativity is stifled and the appetite subdued. The kitchen is the main room in which to recognize and honour our connection to nature; by using natural materials to create the kitchen itself, this bond is reaffirmed.

The solidity of stone, the warm, giving nature of linoleum or cork and the ancient calming influence of wood have the effect of slowing us down from the mental rat-race that directs most of our lives. This allows us to refocus our attention on the spiritual and physical sustenance that food brings to our holistic wellbeing. Good ergonomic design will allow the physical body to be adequately supported but the appropriateness of the finishing texture is always an important consideration, as it is this that provides the sensory envelope necessary for true comfort.

Above all, you want your home to make you feel safe and supported. The trick is to decide on the purpose of a room and then how you wish to experience it. This is not a working environment, an art gallery, a museum or a show home: this is your place of refuge and it should yield to you as you return for rest and recuperation. Wooden (or, worse still, wrought iron) indoor staircases may look attractive but will cost stress in terms of noise and the fear of falling. Similarly, precariously displayed works of art, white or pale plain furnishings or designs that simply require too much care, will all detract from the primary role of the home which is to look after you. A bedroom should be soft and yielding, wrapping a loving embrace around you as you fall into a happy, secure sleep. A kitchen should be inspirational yet grounding, practical and easy to keep clean yet also warming to heart and mind. A dining room should encourage those dining to linger, relishing both their food and the company. By making sure that the textures and surfaces in your home support you physically and emotionally, you will dramatically enhance your experience of it, so think which materials inspire these moods as you begin to plan each room.

Textiles are a relatively cheap and easy way of re-interpreting a room on a seasonal basis. By having two sets of interchangeable soft furnishings, not only is their life-span increased but the homeowner also benefits from the renewed energy invoked by the act of changeover. Cotton and hemp/cotton mixes, cheesecloth, linen and voile are perfect for the spring and summer months when curtains, cushions, throws and rugs need to be light in weight, easy to wash if taken on picnics or into the garden, and even re-dyed if the Sun fades them too much. Wool, velvet, felt and faux fur, on the other hand, are an expensive investment best shielded from strong sunlight and the wear and tear of summer's exuberance.

As well as being a factor in itself, texture brings a second dimension to the design statement implied by colour. Different materials will push any given hue further towards a particular sensation: warm, cool, hot, cold, hard, absorbing, masculine or feminine. This means that a scheme based on the neutral palette will differ in temperature depending on whether your flooring is creamy sandstone tiling or a soft, naturally-coloured woollen carpet. Compare rich red velvet to wispy, ruby-coloured muslin: both are evocative, but one is heavy and sensuous, the other light and flirtatious. Combining wool with velvet will warm an interior whatever the colour choice, but if hot colours are then added to the mix, cosy may inadvertently become claustrophobic, especially if the room faces south. A cool blue bathroom will quickly become a cold, unyielding environment when the hard surfaces of chrome, tiles and concrete are added; compensate by adding the fluffiest towels, the softest lighting and the verdancy of moisture-loving plants. Alternatively, a hot room can be cooled by fresh, flat materials such as linen, silk, stone and wood.

Finally, remember that texture can be used in conjunction with colour to create rooms which are gender-harmonized. A bedroom that is painted pink would feel overly-feminine if it were furnished in fluffy fabrics and deep pile carpets. However, teaming the pink paintwork with dark wood floors, crisp white linens and simple, clean-lined furniture would make the room more balanced. Similarly, a blue bedroom can be made to feel less boyish by incorporating multi-layered fabrics, ornate furnishings and pretty patterns.

SCENT

The olfactory nerves situated in the nose are responsible for transporting smell information to the brain. Our own smell is our calling card and, whether we wish consciously to admit it or not, is as least as fundamental to our being as how we look or what we say. The powerful pheromones that each and every one of us release allow us to assess fairly accurately whether someone is a threat or a possible mate, and whether we should engage with them or take flight. We all exude and respond to the very specific information carried by these olfactory teasers, so take a moment to consider what you are saying about yourself to the world right now. Are you exuding fear or love? Aggression or submissiveness? Health or ill-health?

Scent and its slightly less appealing partner smell are all around us; for our purposes within the home, these can be divided into those which are unpleasant, those which are pleasant and those which are therapeutic. Our brains tend to focus their attention on a particular smell for a very limited period and, once again, this is for reasons of survival. However, that does not mean that the influence of a given smell subsides after such a time. Just because our brains choose to disregard a smell, having established its nature, its influence doesn't stop and this is particularly worth remembering with regard to unpleasant smells. As far as these are concerned, you have to act on logic rather than instinct. You may not notice the bin, the cat litter, the dog's blankets or last night's dinner but anyone entering your home will.

So keep on top of the causes of any potential olfactory offence by opening the window, doing the washing up, washing those blankets and re-siting the cat litter outside. Do not rely on commercial odour neutralizers; most work by using synthetic chemicals to coat the sensors in your nose, depriving you of the ability to detect the smell while the smell still remains. Any synthetic smells, whether from perfume, room deodorizers, air fresheners, cleaning agents or toiletries, simply mask the original smell and contain yet more chemicals which our bodies don't need.

Pleasant smells are obviously to be encouraged but, again, be aware of the screening process that our brains employ. The lovely bunch of flowers you bought last week may still look beautiful but what's that slightly vegetable smell your friend can notice? Could it be the odour of rotting stalks in foetid water?

For smells to have any therapeutic benefit, they must come from a natural, living source such as flowers, fruits, herbs and seeds. The ability of plants and their oils to promote and preserve health was noted by ancient civilizations as geographically and culturally diverse as Mesopotamia, China and Egypt. Having realized that, out of all the professions, it was the perfume makers who were seemingly immune to often highly-contagious diseases, the power of plants to cure and prevent illness began to be documented. By the 16th century, alchemists were still searching for a fifth element which they believed pervaded all things spiritual and earthly: the quintessence of life. The phrase summed up the highly-refined and therapeutically potent oils that were being extracted from plants; in time, these came to be known as 'essence' or 'essential oils'. From the ancient Egyptians (who used oils to combat depression) to the modern health resorts found nestling in the oil-drenched atmosphere of the Swiss pine forests, the energy encapsulated in the molecules of these natural aromas has been harnessed for the good of humankind, animals and even plants themselves. Full use of this natural bonanza can also be taken to create a pleasing and healthy home.

The powerful physiological process which these oils initiate begins when their concentrated charge of bio-electrical energy is absorbed through the skin and the olfactory nerves in the nose and from there passes into every cell and tissue of the body. Essential oils have the ability to cleanse, heal, reduce inflammation, kill bacteria, boost immunity, relax, revitalize, uplift and calm, all without leaving any harmful residue in the body.

However, they are extremely concentrated and, though natural and (in the main) non-toxic, they must be used with care, stored safely and not used on young children or animals without professional guidance. The essential oil of oregano, for instance, is 26 times more powerful an antiseptic than phenol, the main ingredient in many commercial cleansing products. If possible, use organic oils, especially when cooking. The following oils are recommended as a starter kit but they must be used in diluted form either in a carrier oil (such as sweet almond), in a heat diffuser, in the bath or inhaled as a vapour. Once diluted, patch tests are advisable in case of the unlikely event of an allergic reaction. These cautions noted, there are many ways in which these oils can be utilized to enhance our own health, beauty and cleanliness, whilst at the same time giving our spirits a boost through the delightful smells that fill our homes and senses.

GERANIUM: a wonderful mood-enhancer. Put six drops in an oil burner to help harmonize extremes of both emotional and physical conditions and/or use the same amount diluted in an eggcup full of sweet almond oil to massage the body back into a state of balance. The antiseptic and astringent qualities of this oil make it useful for combination-skin: add one or two drops to preparations such as face-packs and scrubs.

LEMON: you'll never be short of lemons as long as you have a bottle of this oil in the house. Add two or three drops to your regular cooking or salad oil to bring the flavour and goodness of lemons to your meal. Six drops used in a house plant sprayer will keep the atmosphere in your home pleasingly fresh. Two drops in warm water with honey will help to relieve a cold while one drop in plain warm water will aid digestion. One drop added to your facial scrub will tone the skin and three or four drops in the bath will stimulate the immune system.

CHAMOMILE: is antispasmodic, an analgesic and an anti-inflammatory oil, as suggested by the soothing blue colour of German chamomile. Use six drops in the bath or in a heat diffuser to calm a body overheated by fever, pain or emotional anxiety. The gentler Roman chamomile is particularly beneficial if you have children, but use only three to four drops in an eggcup full of massage oil or in a diffuser fitted around a light bulb.

LAVENDER: the all-round healing oil. One or two drops of this oil can be used neat on burns, wounds and bruises. It is anti-inflammatory and antiseptic and it encourages cells to regenerate more rapidly, allowing wounds to heal more quickly. It is soothing to heat in both the body and the mind.

TEA TREE: The only other oil which can safely be used neat on the skin. Its antiseptic and anti-fungal properties are invaluable to the family during the annual cold season, when four drops can be added to a warm bath or inhaled from a steamy bowl of water. Its ability to dissolve pus can cleanse a wound and, at the same time, provide a tonic to a run-down immune system.

SOUND

Around 3000 years ago, priests from the Hindu faith wrote down the sacred scriptures that are collectively known as the *Veda*. These ancient hymns were written in Sanskrit and took the form of chants, tunes, prayers and formulae which resonated with the threads or *sutras* of the cosmos. Later, Ancient Egyptian philosophers intuited a connection between music and the heavens and, under the conviction that a celestial symphony was being eternally played out by the movement of the planets, they assigned each of the seven musical notes a planetary twin. Now, at the beginning of the 21st century, physicists still struggling to uncover 'a theory of everything' believe that the fundamental building blocks of the universe are not point-like particles but string-like substances which resonate in a ten-dimensional form as yet beyond our comprehension. This mathematical theory, known as Superstring, theorizes that it is vibration that underpins the existence of both the tangible world and worlds that are as yet indiscernible. Whether Superstring does turn out to be the unifying theory of the cosmos is yet to be seen, but what is known is that where there is vibration, there is resonance and where there is resonance, there is the potential for either harmony or discord.

When creating a holistically-pleasing home, it is essential to pay attention to the sounds emanating from within it and to ensure that they are as harmonizing as possible. Certain sounds have an inherently soothing quality and these have been used very successfully as a form of therapy for the treatment of psychological imbalances.

Other sounds, however, seem to jangle at the nerves, triggering imbalance. The difference between the two is more than simply a matter of taste; it is not only the *type* of sound that determines its effect upon us, but also our *relationship* to its cause. The filtering system employed by the brain to manage sensory input allows us to ignore safe or expected sound, paying attention only to that which signals change or danger. This same filtration system permits us to ignore the mass clamour of a social gathering but still to hear our own name mentioned across the room as if it is being hailed through a loud speaker. Whether or not noise becomes truly offensive depends on our relationship with the offender and how much control we have over the situation.

If, for example, the Council has written to give notice of six weeks of repair work outside your house, the situation will be less stressful than if you have had no warning and no idea when it may terminate. Similarly, if householders give adequate warning of any particularly disruptive parties or D.I.Y, neighbours are offered the chance to take evasive action, meaning that the disturbance will be more readily tolerated. Unfortunately, as population densities increase, the potential for sound to become a polluter is increasing. Inadequate sound insulation and our 24/7 lifestyles, combined with ever more powerful sound systems, make intrusive noise a major cause of neighbourly discord. Finally, laws are coming into effect which will require all new buildings and conversions to meet performance specifications which include an insistence on adequate sound insulation. Meanwhile, for those of us ensconced in existing buildings, there is much that can be done to minimize noise pollution both from external sources as well as from inside our own home.

There are various ways in which noise travels: through the air; as impact, either overhead or on walls and through transmission along the ground or floor surface. Generally, it's a combination of all three but, whatever the outside is doing, the first step to resolving noise pollution is to tackle that which comes from within the home itself.

Often dismissed as an unavoidable by-product of the natural goings-on in and around a home, sound is frequently an ignored component of home design. The trend for knocking down walls to create a spacious kitchen/dining area can result in a cavernous expanse which, if furnished with hard flooring and wooden blinds, will act as a sound-box amplifying every little noise. If you have such a room, the addition of curtains, carpets and soft furnishings will help to act as a baffle to the clatter of cutlery, china and chat. If you are determined to have hard flooring, do at least consider carpeting the stairs and main walkways in order to reduce the impact of footfall. If you are lucky enough to have the space, investing in the creation of a utility area allows noisy appliances such as the refrigerator, washing machine or dishwasher to go about their business whilst leaving the kitchen area undisturbed. That said, most modern kitchens are now home to an array of electrical equipment not known to previous generations: food mixers, juicers, liquidizers and extractor fans, to name but a few. Keeping an objective eye on just how many gadgets you really need means that you can monitor overall levels of noise pollution. For all other appliances, make sure that they are fully turned off when not in use in order to eliminate the low-level hum associated with stand-by mode. As a further step, take the time to oil creaking doors, fix dripping taps and bleed radiators and, in so doing, significantly reduce the clatter that now afflicts many homes in much the same way as clutter does.

When noise comes in from an external source over which you have no control, screening is the solution. This involves the absorption, blocking or baffling of sound vibrations; once again, simple steps make quite a difference. For many people, double-glazing is the most obvious (although environmentally expensive) answer but, by simply ensuring that doors, windows and their frames fit properly, incoming disturbance can be significantly reduced. If noise through walls is a problem, putting up shelves lined with books can act as an attractive baffle and, in extreme cases, acoustic insulation quilting can be wall-mounted behind plasterboard to create a relatively cost-effective solution. If the problem is a busy road, sand placed under a ground floor will reduce the impact of noise vibration. Using thickly-padded curtains to cover windows and doorways will further muffle sound as well as reducing heat loss in winter. Some of the most intrusive noise pollution comes from overhead neighbours and, unfortunately, this can be the most difficult and expensive to eliminate. If they cannot be persuaded to put down carpets and rugs, the only option may be to install a false ceiling, one that complies with professional specifications for noise reduction.

Some noises may seem to be natural or harmonious but can still cause offence. Metal wind ornaments clanging around in the breeze are more crime than chime, while a continuous stream of water can be more reminiscent of a tap left running than a babbling brook. Better to open a window on to an environment that attracts songbirds to splash in a birdbath, while trees and grasses shimmer and rustle in the breeze. Always try to ensure that the sounds filling your home are the ones that heal rather than harass but, above all, remember that, as far as both you and your neighbour are concerned, it is silence that is truly golden.

Essential Elements

The elements of air, water, fire and Earth form the fundamental building blocks of our existence. Without air we cannot breathe, without water we dehydrate, we need Earth's nourishment for our bodies and fire's warmth for the soul. A successful home will pay homage to these base elements, reminding us of the simplicity of our true selves, as opposed to the man-made complexities of modern existence. Their presence also symbolizes our connection to that most primal of energies, the planet herself. With her fiery core, deep oceans and boundless sky, the elements forge a link between ourselves in the here and now and the very moment the Earth was created. We are both a product of that ancient combustion of raw energy and the relevance of these elements to our physical and emotional wellbeing is as fundamental today as it has always been.

On a physiological level, oxygen feeds our blood whilst minerals from the Earth form the building blocks of our cells and tissues. Water permeates each and every cell, allowing the absorption of nutrients and the expulsion of waste. Fire flows as electricity through our nerves and fibres, allowing messages to be sent around the body at lightning speed. The elements are used to describe various personality types; some people are earthy while others both attract and scare us with their fiery temperament. Another still may be said to have their head in the clouds, or to possess a personality that is deep and unfathomable. The ancient art of astrology separates us into elemental signs and many health systems, including the Ayurvedic and homeopathic, use the elements to categorize body-types and so prescribe appropriate healing treatments. When truly at ease, one is said to be in one's element and it is then that inspiration and vision seem to come most effortlessly. Colours, materials and imagery all carry an inherent elemental nature; by becoming aware of this, a balanced foundation can be ensured within the home which will allow creativity to blossom.

EARTH

We draw energy from deep within the Earth, through the nourishment that is gained from its harvest to the materials that are used to build our houses and possessions. Our sense of who we are draws its meaning from the path we choose to walk; it is therefore essential to our good health that we feel grounded and sure under foot. *Querencia* is an Old Spanish word meaning 'the place on Earth from which the heart draws strength'. Only by searching for and finding our true *querencia* can we put down energetic roots and then, just like the Great Redwood trees themselves, truly begin to grow.

Within the home, there are a number of ways in which to ensure our connection to Earth's grounding energy, beginning with the paint on the walls. Originally, paint was derived from mineral pigments such as ochre, sienna or terre verte and, today, many paint-manufacturing companies are returning to these natural resources to produce colours which have a depth not only of colour but also of character. With names such as Venetian pink and Oxford ochre, these original Earth pigments evoke the hills of Tuscany and the wall-washes of old English cottages. Raw and burnt umber, Indian red, lamp black, ochre, green Earth, raw and burnt sienna all have a very grounding quality, perfectly suited to the simplicity and robustness of Shaker and ethnic designs. They can also be used to bring a warmth and complexity to modern interiors by creating schemes that come alive as the light plays on the contrasting surfaces. Other colours are more reminiscent of Earth's riches, such as the jewel-like tones of ruby, sapphire, amethyst and emerald, but both palettes have real resonance, making them a far more interesting choice than the tinnier hues of sugar pink or acidic green that come into occasional fashion. It's easy to tire of bright, zany colours but they can be successfully used if incorporated as highlights against a backdrop of neutral, earthy mainstays. By teaming them with natural fibres such as unbleached linens or cottons and textures such as wood, rattan and seagrass an earthy contrast is incorporated which brings balance to an otherwise overly-stimulating scheme. If you are feeling adventurous, many workshops are held to teach the art of vegetable dyeing, which produces a much more subtle colour tint, perfectly suited to the natural home.

When it comes to filling our homes, Earth's energy is represented in many ways. Anything from a bunch of flowers to a pair of oversized stone candlesticks honours her for her benevolence. Whether it's a bone china tea set brought out to mark a special occasion or simply the colour and nutrition found in a bowl of fruit, the element of Earth acts to ground and support us. At a time of insecurity, a beautiful stone sculpture can help to bring the weighty reassurance that is needed. Or, should the preciousness of life seem temporarily lost, a carefully-chosen crystal may re-ignite the sparkle in your eye.

Remember though that the Earth is not an endless, private store cupboard put there for our benefit only. One can draw strength, but should also take the opportunity to give back by ensuring that our planet is treated with the respect she deserves. One of the best ways of doing this is, wherever possible, to allow only natural materials into your home. Use wood certified as coming from carefully managed forests, rather than chemical-ridden MDF. Use only low VOC or preferably non-toxic paints. Seek out natural alternatives to the vast array of chemicals on offer, be it for the home or for yourself.

Non-toxic, renewable products, chemical-free cleaning, organic food and non-chemical based healthcare all honour the planet and its complex ecosystem, so do yourself and all of Earth's creatures a favour and banish those environmental and health-damaging chemicals once and for all.

Of course, whilst Earth is so dependably there to support us, it is also capable of smothering us. If left unchecked by a balance of other energy, we could become literally Earth-bound; to prevent us from becoming stuck in the proverbial rut, it is essential to incorporate some of life's other energies, to lift our spirits and allow us to soar.

FIRE

Whereas the Earth element provides a firm foundation from which to begin, fire is concerned with inspiration. It is both the spark that ignites our imagination and the finishing touch that brings a home or a setting to life.

The presence of real fire gives magic to any setting and all the main festivals, both religious and secular, make use of candles to emphasize this sense of being special. Within the home whether taking a bath, sharing a meal, relaxing alone or with friends candlelight immediately draws us into its intimacy. Any otherwise mundane event takes on the feeling of an occasion; it becomes special time and we become special with it. When sitting before a real fire be it a fireplace, outside watching a bonfire, or even gathered around a barbecue our evolutionary past stirs within us, each flame a reminder of the transience of our time, burning most brightly before it flickers and dies. It is this ability to shed light on our deepest thoughts and feelings which means that fire's absence leaves us physically and emotionally in the dark. Everyone needs fire in their lives, but its unpredictable nature and potential for destruction means that it demands our respect in a way in which no other element does. The life-giving heat and light that emanate from our wonderful Sun are equally capable of causing drought, famine and devastating fires. By unleashing instantaneous volcanic mayhem, fire can rip through our sure Earth and destroy all in its path. This awesome power holds a fascination from which it is hard to turn away. Unable to be touched or held, the burning flame remains an elusive beacon, illuminating the soul, inspiring us to dream and ponder. It is the element of fire that can drive away fear, bring inspiration to our hearts and a welcoming warmth to our homes.

The fire has always been an integral part of the home and it is still relied upon today to provide warmth, light and cooked food. If you are lucky enough to own a working fireplace, make sure that the chimney is properly lined and regularly swept so that the fire draws efficiently. Since the advent of gas and electricity, cleaner, more efficient forms of heating have replaced many working fireplaces but you can still honour fire's energy by creating a focus. This could take the form of a sacred heart within the home, where precious objects are brought together, either where the fire would be or in another likely spot. Whether or not a fireplace is present, our instinct to huddle remains so ingrained that, inevitably, there continues to be a focus of communal attention: the television. Like a real fire, television can draw a family together but it can also preclude conversation and sharing. By using the colours of fire, we can keep communal rooms welcoming even when the television isn't on, encouraging the family to gather together whenever possible. A central rug of the richest tones of gold, red or orange will bring focus to a sitting room, whilst similar colours employed as a table dressing have the effect of drawing everyone in, encouraging the sharing of thoughts and feelings, much as would have happened around a campfire.

Another way to evoke fire's sparkle is through the use of coloured glass and crystal. Any light reflecting on these surfaces becomes reminiscent of the playfulness of the living flame, reminding us of the truly dynamic nature of fire. Using these objects in the presence of candles or firelight will bring instant magic to any setting: refracting, reflecting and polarizing the energy, incandescent with possibility.

Finally, fire's energy can be used to concentrate those thoughts which we are not ready to share. For centuries, the simple white candle has been a symbol of purity of thought and spirit, lit by people of all faiths to enhance meditative time and to connect with the higher truth of their beliefs. Within the home, such a candle may be lit whenever clarity is needed or peace sought. For the flame is above all concerned with truth. It is not about show, for all its brilliant glory. It is about the inner light which burns so brightly within each of us, if only we have the courage to let it shine.

WATER

As with the all the elements, water has a dual role as both giver and taker of life. This means that, whilst we depend on water for survival, it also has the capacity to overwhelm and drown us. Water will soothe a fevered brow or refresh the weary traveller but many people find that, when facing the vastness of the open sea, water begins to evoke a different, somewhat more anxious response. Over 70% of the planet is water, yet more is known about deep space than about the deep sea. The tidal flow of the great oceans is governed by the massive influence of the Moon yet her impact on the human body, which contains a similar proportion of water, remains largely ignored. Each person begins life in a watery haven, just as our species began life in the sea and, after all the thousands of years of our evolution, the mineral composition of our own blood plasma is almost identical to the seawater from which we emerged.

Although our bodies are more water than flesh and blood, if you cut the skin you do not find water as such, rather it is the carrier that facilitates our physical being. Whatever our body's molecular make-up may be, water carries with it the resonance of our evolutionary journey, of all that informs our being, the transmitter of our Soul.

A simple glance at house plants left un-watered graphically illustrates what happens when our bodies are left to dehydrate; what may be less obvious are the emotional repercussions. It is said that the key to a less stressful life is to learn to go with the flow, but how can we expect to flow if 70% of our body is crying out for lubrication? It is all too easy to become literally stuck, frustrated in life or relationships and blocked from attaining goals and desires. But the fluid nature of water and its ability to transmute into ice, steam, frost and snow reminds us that nothing in this life is fixed or carved in stone. A river or glacier cutting through sheer rock illustrates how powerful this force for change can be; just as water finds its course, so we will find ours.

With regard to water in the home, the obvious place to start is the bathroom. There is a temptation to give bathrooms a watery feel by painting the room in various shades of blue. However, this is to misinterpret our relationship with water; the inherent coolness of the blue can make us feel cold, more reminiscent of being adrift in high seas than supported by warm, maternal waters. It is far better to create a supportive scheme which uses the colours of coral, sand and shells along with soft lighting, fragrant oils and warm, yielding textures. Doing so allows us to give substance to that which contains the water (i.e. the bathroom) then, as you experience your watery retreat, be it a bath or shower, your eyes can gaze on the nearness of that which we all hope to reach: the shore.

After a day spent surrounded by computers, artificial lighting, machinery and traffic, all of our stresses cling to us like an irritable rash. What is happening on a physiological level is that the atoms in our bodies have become positively charged by their proximity to so much electricity and metal, so becoming slothful and lacking in energy. A bath or shower will literally turn your atomic energy around for you, negatively ionizing this electrical charge and causing your atoms to become full of vim and vigour instead. This is the reason why we always feel better by the sea or a tumbling river. By using water to bring our physical bodies back to an optimum state of wellbeing, our emotional selves can concentrate on their true purpose, which is not to react but to create.

In addition to its therapeutic actions of hydration, cleansing and ionizing, water can also be playful, meditative and creative. A paddling pool will always provide fun for children of all ages, whilst a bath can be both an aid to relaxation and a therapeutic warm-up to a busy day. A water feature can bring with it either a contemplative stillness or the tumbling energy of a babbling brook. Either will become an instant attraction to passing birds, insects and even animals, encouraging their vibrant energy into the home and garden environment. Pictures, collages, stencils and motifs can all be used to bring water's energy into our homes, but remember to use imagery wisely. For some the sea can induce intense anxiety, where feelings of awe at the ocean's immensity and fear of the unknown induce a sort of claustrophobia and agoraphobia combined. The colour blue exacerbates these feelings, appearing as it does to recede. Always be particularly careful when painting murals in children's rooms and ensure that the overall effect is safe and grounded rather than lost at sea.

In these days of disappearing natural resources, it would not be responsible to recommend the pillaging of our beaches for shells and driftwood with which to decorate our homes. There are many who already do possess such a collection; if this is the case for you, use these treasures of the deep as a reminder of the ocean's mystery and preciousness. The seas are dying before our eyes; the impact that this is going to have in the very near future is catastrophic. Always be responsible towards the sea in the products and produce that you buy and make sure that you, your laundry and your dishes are washed in water-friendly products only.

The ability to flow through life's rocky course means that we reach our destination as smoothly as possible. This whole notion of flow links us to our final element: that of the air.

AIR

Our planet's precisely-balanced mixture of gases forms the final piece of the puzzle that allows life on Earth to flourish. As with all of the elements, air has its destructive side. Tornadoes, hurricanes or cyclones: high winds can sweep away entire settlements, leaving a path of devastation as precise as that of any cutting tool. As ever, it is a case of the gentlest touch being the breath of life, the most ferocious being the kiss of death.

Air is associated with mental capacity; it is said that a clear head or headspace is needed in order to think rationally, whilst fresh air is known to blow the cobwebs away, clearing mental or emotional agues. In folklore, wind was recognized as a harbinger of what's to come. It was said to bring a change of fortunes and depending on the direction of the wind, that fortune may be good or bad. So, whereas water symbolizes the mystery of the unseen (i.e. our spirit), air symbolizes all of life's possibilities, i.e. our potential.

The continual movement of air allows seeds to colonize new areas, brings information to the animal kingdom and keeps the British obsessed with the weather in order to plan the weekend. Yet, such is the pollution from cars and lorries, it is only by going out into real countryside or up into the highest mountain ranges that we begin to appreciate the true nature of this element. Sadly, rather than taking serious steps to cut down on pollution, our tendency is to seal ourselves off from the outside world with double glazing, extractor fans and walled-up chimneys. Instead, we should be creating a world that allows us to throw open the windows and breathe in all that life has to offer, for to breathe in is literally to 'inspire'.

As usual, the problem is less complicated than we might like to pretend. Walking or cycling not only cuts down on pollution but also on the likelihood of getting osteoporosis, heart disease, obesity, cancer and a myriad of other ailments. Time spent outdoors also allows access to that other great health-giver: the Sun. 30 minutes each day spent walking outdoors in the fresh air under full spectrum sunlight will do you far more good physically and emotionally than a once-a-week burn in the gym. It's free, too.

Within the home, access as much fresh air as possible by making sure that there is adequate ventilation and circulation. Ensure that as many windows as possible open but, if you are on the ground floor, think about security, too. It is better to have two smaller windows open and to feel safe than to open one big window which you have to keep an eye on. Encourage airflow by opening windows at the front and back of your home and allowing a through draught. The presence of open chimneys and air vents helps to maintain a balanced internal environment by allowing for a continuous change of air. Ventilation is all-important when it comes to preventing a build-up of fumes; better still, stop fumes at source by having all appliances correctly maintained and by banishing all chemical fluids and sprays.

Ensure that curtains do not encroach on the actual window space any more than is necessary. By keeping window dressings simple and extending the curtain pole or rail beyond the window width, as much air will be allowed to waft in as possible. Fabrics also possess an inherent energy; here, too, air's lightness of being can be emphasized by featherweight fabrics such as muslin, organza, cheesecloth, voile and lace. The flimsiness of these fabrics allows them to waft against the slightest breeze, emphasizing the movement of air.

Make sure that the materials used on the walls and floors of your home are permeable, to allow an exchange of air and moisture. Micro-porous paints and varnishes made from natural ingredients are available from specialist companies both for interior and exterior walls, as are wax finishes for floors and furniture. Using these products will ensure that neither you nor your home's ability to breathe healthily will be compromised.

One of the most popular wind ornaments is the ubiquitous chime. As discussed in the chapter on sound, a certain degree of judiciousness is needed where wind chimes are concerned. The clanging of metal will do nothing for you or your neighbours' nerves and it should be remembered that chimes were originally intended to demarcate different areas of energy inside the home, rather than in the garden at the mercy of every nor'wester that comes in. Bamboo chimes are preferable as they elicit a more harmonious, natural sound, but better still is the rustle of plants on either side of an open window. Of course, the choice of garden plants is endless but not all houseplants tolerate a draught. The simple spider-plant, however, will.

Finally, attempt to maintain a lightness of feel throughout the home generally. It is easy to find oneself weighed down by the sheer number of possessions and the responsibility felt towards them. Remember that it's not what you own that defines you. Even if you are not ready to let go of your things, try to limit how much more you add. You really will feel lighter and freer in a clean, uncluttered home, less encumbered and more energized. Your home should not be spartan (in the sense of the minimalist aesthetic) but neither does it have to be a museum. Life is about the moment: be free enough to grab each one as it comes.

CHAPTER 16

Inspiration

The daily routine that directs most of our lives would soon become hum-drum without the interjection of something a little more dynamic and stimulating. When inspiration bursts upon us, it breaks through the normality of everyday being, animating the imagination and re-igniting our sense of purpose. It is inspiration that prevents our thoughts and actions from becoming mundane, allowing our intuitive creativity a chance to shine.

Rather like breathing itself, inspiration is a question of 'in' and 'out'. We inspire fresh air, which feeds our bodies and minds with all that is new and good. We then expire the used air, expelling all that we have no need of. Life begins with a deep inhalation and ends with a final outward breath. Our excitements are marked by gasps of exclamation, our sadnesses by a procession of sighs. The in-and-out nature of respiration serves as a reminder that the ability to act on inspiration is dependent on having already let go of all that is unhelpful. After all, you cannot take a deep breath without first relaxing your muscles and emptying your lungs. Only by keeping mental channels uncluttered is it possible to recognize the sudden flashes of clarity that are capable of propelling us towards new understanding. Breathing rhythmically and beneficially forms the basis of many meditative techniques, helping to still the mind and provide a literal breathing space from which inspiration can then arise like spring water. The preceding chapters have shown how the various elements of design can be used to support us on a physical and emotional level. But it is also possible to use specially-chosen objects and colours to help lift us out of the daily pattern of our lives, to refocus our frequently chaotic thoughts and excite our lust for all that life has to offer.

The place to start is the point of entry and exit: the front door. This gateway to our home is more than just a physical barrier: it is the point where public space becomes private domain, the moment at which we physically and metaphorically take our coats off and begin to relax. It is this act of relaxation that helps to free us from the emotional tangles of the day, allowing us to reconnect with our true selves. By choosing a colour that truly inspires you, your front door will sing out and become a welcome home symbol to yourself and a calling card to outsiders. By maintaining the frame, fittings and fixtures to the highest standard possible, you can ensure that your door speaks as an ambassador for your home, a signpost of what visitors can expect inside. Sometimes, the front door permits itself to be overlooked, allowing no positive change in us emotionally or physically, but this is to miss out on a wonderful opportunity for emotional catharsis.

Metaphorically, the entrance to our homes can be seen as the keyhole to our true being; investing in this portal is investing in our sense of self.

The first step to take is to ascertain the effectiveness of the door. Does it work? Check for good locks and a draught-proof fit, ease of opening and closing, lack of squeak and a letterbox that won't take off the postman's hand. Secondly, consider sympathy. Is the style of the door in keeping with the architecture of the house? If not, it will jar which means that, on some level, so will you. And what about its character? If the windows are the eyes of the house, the door is definitely the mouth. Is yours smiling or sad, enticing or toothless?

The other point to consider is the material from which the door is made. There are a worrying number of PVC doors out there and these should be resisted as firmly as PVC windows. Apart from carrying high environmental costs, they completely ignore the importance of the energetic nature inherent in natural materials. Poly-Vinyl Chloride is synthetic and therefore energetically dead. Wood (taken from sustainable resources only), on the other hand, is a natural material that has been harvested to give us warmth and shelter for thousands of years: no other material can match it. In its pre-felled state, wood plunges its roots deep down into the Earth and reaches up into the skies above, forming the link between our Earth-bound physicality and our sky-bound spirit. Remember that it is wood that is chosen as the carrier for our final journey, facilitating our transition from this world into the next. It is therefore entirely appropriate that it should also be used as the portal between the external and internal worlds of the here and now.

The colour we choose for our front door speaks volumes. Many people opt for the safety of black or non-committal white. These can be good choices, as black is said to absorb negative vibrations whilst white deflects them, but these colours are better used on the frame rather than on the door itself, for here there is scope to be far more imaginative. Some colours have cultural associations; the Native Americans and the people of the eastern Mediterranean both use turquoise to ornament an entrance because it is seen as protective, whilst yellow is seen as auspicious by the followers of Feng Shui. There is no right or wrong colour for a front door but it should be a colour that inspires you. Of course, this may be harder to settle on if you are a family of five or a group of housemates but the fact that you have sought each other out means that there must be some common ground somewhere. It might be that you choose to show off your diversity by having an eccentric decoration, but be careful that this appeals to all of you and not just to the dominant character. Alternatively, a plain door can be enhanced by planting flowers and shrubs around the entrance, allowing a more diverse colour energy into the area, as well as a pleasing fragrance. Coloured glass incorporated into the door or frame can look lovely when done well and is another way to attract colour energy into your home. The important thing is to use a colour that you love. That way, every time you set eyes upon your front door, your spirits will lift and you'll enter your home with a lighter heart.

Hopefully, all of the colours and objects in your home will be inspirational to some degree; what they should be inspiring is love, happiness, fond memories, self-worth and respect for life. The mementoes, artwork, artefacts, photographs and certificates of achievement with which we surround ourselves not only track our development so far but also signpost the way forward, engendering the possibility of future achievements. Anything that triggers irritation, anger, pain or doubt should be thrown out (or recycled) with the other rubbish as it is just not needed. A useful exercise involves looking at everything you own and noting your honest reaction to each item. This is quite an undertaking, but it is not necessary to cover the whole house in an afternoon. Just get into the habit of questioning what you have about you and then acting on your responses. The fact that you have actively thought about the objects with which you surround yourself will be an inspiration in itself.

Nature, especially human nature, seems to abhor a void but if you are lucky enough to have space in your home, treasure it and devote it to maintaining your internal equilibrium or headspace. Whether to facilitate gentle exercise, relaxation or meditation, a dedicated space is a valuable investment in health. A tidy, uncluttered bedroom could provide space for daily meditation or room enough for yoga. Alternatively, a comfortable chair looking out over a natural vista will offer rest to a tired body and a contemplative view to a fraught mind. The important thing is to have access to natural light and for the space to feel devoted. Incorporating a simple, single object of inspiration such as a candle, a meditative mandala or yantra painting will bring focus, whether you are creating art or simply peace of mind.

The area in which most people seem to feel the need for a little inspiration is work. For many, this takes place away from home but, wherever it happens, take the time to assess your space and decide how you can foster a little joy in it. Even if you share an open-plan office space with twenty others, you can still bring a little personal booster into the frame, uplifting your spirits and bolstering your sense of you-ness. A simple plant is a good start as not only will it connect you to nature but it sends out the subtle reminder that life isn't all about work and neither will the world stop turning if work stops. It also brings with it the energy of growth, rebirth and regeneration which is so necessary to smart-working practice. If you have a free hand to decorate as you wish, so much the better. Begin by making the space workable then bring in something that excites your imagination and creativity. Think about what you need to make your working life productive and fulfilling. Is it quiet reflection or something more dynamic? Limit yourself to one or two choices, any more than that and the space will feel crowded, stifling the flow of creativity. Whether at work or at home, always remember that these chosen items can and should be changed according to your energies, maybe on a seasonal basis or to reflect the ebb and flow of your working or personal life. If not, they will lose their ability to inspire, cease to be noticed and simply become clutter.

CHAPTER 17

❁ ❁ ❁   # Connection   ❁ ❁ ❁

Our re-awakening to this interaction with our homes has been accelerated in the last few years by the arrival on Western shores of the ancient Chinese art of geomancy. After the materialism of the 1980s, many were left feeling that something was missing from the trite world we had created and it was hoped that Feng Shui, as this art is known, might just fill the void. For those unaware of the principles behind Feng Shui, here is an exceedingly brief introduction.

Feng Shui literally means 'wind and water' and the essence of its philosophy is harmony and flow. Feng Shui Masters look at the spaces in which people live and work and relate them to what is termed the 'Bagua'. This is also known as the 'magic square' and was originally inspired by the markings on the shell of a tortoise. The separate areas within the Bagua relate specifically to different aspects of nature: Heaven, Earth, Fire, Water, Mountain, Lake, Wind and Thunder, with the Yin-Yang symbol representing Unity in the centre. By correctly imposing this Bagua on to the floor-plan of a given space, exponents believe that all aspects of the occupant's reality are reflected back at them. By placing symbolic cures and enhancements in the relevant areas, Feng Shui practitioners believe that it is possible to manifest change in the related areas of the occupant's life.

Whilst Feng Shui makes use of several universal truths, the fact is that such personal changes will only manifest when the individual truly, fundamentally wills it to be so. Unfortunately, Feng Shui has suffered on Western shores because it is a practice alien to the people of this culture and, as long as we continue to use it in the same way that we use many other supposed panaceas (such as pills, money and faux faith), it will never help us to achieve the liberation and healing we crave. This sticking-plaster approach, one that sees individuals hand over what are often significant amounts of money in order for someone else to do the work simply won't help unless we believe in the deepest recesses of our hearts and minds that it will. That is why placebos work and self-denial doesn't.

Only by opening up to the reality behind our existence is it possible to find the peace that allows for real growth. All the complexities of 21st century survival eventually distil down to the same unchanging truth: that we are totally connected to and dependent upon Nature. Respecting and enhancing this connection is the key to all else, including the health, success and longevity both of ourselves as individuals and the species as a whole. As many ancient cultures found to their cost, once mankind seeks to go outside the delicate balance of nature, problems begin to occur. Civilizations as sophisticated and complex as the Mayans of Central America, or even the mighty

Roman Empire, suffered catastrophic and often sudden declines in their fortunes, despite their fiscal wealth and power, because of their increasingly contemptuous treatment of the environment, animals and their fellow human beings. The arrogance which accompanies humankind's apparent ascendancy is, in fact, the precursor to its own fall as problems of soil erosion, rampant disease, corruption and indolence combine to lead to the demise, decay and ultimately death of that particular society.

The key to sustainability is balance: day and night, activity and rest, action and reaction. Everything has an opposite and equal force that acts as a counter-balance, with no one energy allowed to dominate for long before the harmonizing input of an opposing energy comes along to restore equilibrium. It is this that creates the cyclical nature of our world, where all aspects of life are caught up in an unending cycle of growth, rest and regeneration, each part essential to the continuation of both the individual element and of the ecosystem as a whole. A perfect demonstration of this is seen in the life-cycle of a flowering plant. From a single seed, a fully-developed plant arises, attracting insects that facilitate the pollination process and grazing animals that not only gain nourishment from the plant but also leave their droppings to add nutrients to the soil around it. Provided that at least one flower is able to set seed, the plant can ensure the procreation of its species both locally and also in new areas thanks to passing birds, animals and the elements. The original flower eventually withers, its falling leaves adding to the layer of humus that enriches the soil for future generations: an endlessly sustainable cycle of creation.

Then there is humankind. Not content merely to raise more human seedlings, we seek to exploit our time on this Earth with no thought to the future that lies beyond our own demise. It was this wilful short-sightedness which convinced us that it was possible to grow the same crops on the same patch of Earth without suffering a weakening of both the plant and the soil. Our ready belief in chemical fertilizers blinded us to knowledge acquired from thousands of years of sustainable cultivation, with the entirely predictable result that our soil is now utterly depleted in the full range of nutrients vital to the health of the plant. Not only is this bad news for the plant, it is bad news for those dependent on the plant as a crop, with both now becoming nutritionally impoverished and therefore more susceptible to ill-health. If the scenario continues unchecked, the final outcome for both is death. At that point, the land will lie fallow until a less fussy plant comes along and colonizes it, so beginning the cycle of rebirth, though possibly without the attendant human. In just the same way, we cannot defy nature by taking animals out of their natural environment and social groups and expect no alteration in their physiology and behaviour. Whether they are incarcerated in research laboratories or in intensive farms, the fear and pain which they experience on a daily basis causes exactly the same reaction in them as it would in us: susceptibility to disease and weight-loss, thereby invalidating the two reasons we give for putting them there in the first place. Nor can we interfere with a hormonal system that has taken billions of years to evolve and think there will be no come-back. Such is our oestrogen-over-load (thanks to the interference of the chemical hormone-disrupters routinely added to our food crops and livestock) that problems such as breast, endometrial, ovarian, testicular and prostate cancer are becoming ever more prevalent at an ever younger age. The human race is becoming literally disease-ridden, just like the animals and environment which we seek to exploit.

Just as the whole health of any organism is dependent on the correct functioning of all its individual cells, so the health of the planet is dependent upon the optimal input of each individual component. The holistic nature of the Universe dictates that, providing individual cells, organisms or ecosystems are working efficiently, on mass they will begin to work coherently. When this happens, the good of the whole is ensured. For the human race, this principle dictates that it is only by recognizing the implications and repercussions of each and every one of our actions that holistic health can ensue: for the individual, for society and for our planetary ecosystem.

Unfortunately, despite all that history tells us, we are still languishing under the misconception that we are somehow special, above the law of Nature and under the protection of our false gods. We have bought into the belief that the gods favoured us above all others, creating us in their image, when the truth is that we created them in ours. Whichever doctrine is chosen to give form to our lives, be it religious, economic, political or philosophical, the tendency is to go beyond the very natural instinct to survive and to seek instead to dominate.

Christian and Islamic societies, for example, are becoming increasingly polarized despite the fact that both faiths preach tolerance. Communism should have been about the common interest, with each working to the best of their ability and for the benefit of the whole society, but no; it becomes corrupt and gives rise to genocide, that uniquely human achievement. Even the massive, paranoid grip of the communist regime could not be sustained and it eventually collapsed, allowing the rebirth of the capitalist system it had once overthrown. Now, capitalism is seen to be moving away from the ideals of free markets and fair trade to become a rampaging abuse which in the short term ensures that the strong get stronger, whilst the weak get weaker. It too will collapse, as surely as the Sun rises, because it is the nature of things to be cyclical. What the human race needs to be very aware of is the Big Cycle.

Our species is part of a bigger picture, not the mainframe after all and, whether we like it or not, our cycle will come to the point of decay which so necessarily precedes rebirth.

Our society is obsessed with outcomes and end-games but, rather than seeing life simply as a journey towards a specific arrival point (such as promotion, retirement, a dream purchase or even death), it is our conduct on this journey that is going to have the greatest impact on subsequent travellers. Do we lay down a bed of nutritious humus or do we simply take and take until there is nothing left but stony soil and a disease-harbouring cadaver? Continuing to place ourselves outside of nature is the most foolhardy thing that we, as a species, can do but so much has been taken, and so strong is the habit of indulgence, that huge efforts must now be made if the balance is to be restored.

Despite all of our technology and sophistication, our species teeters on the brink of a major cull. This may come from a nuclear explosion triggered by the actions of 'god-fearing' folk or from the more subtle process of wide-scale infertility. What is certain is that our arrogance will facilitate our downfall. Refusal to acknowledge the rights of the rest of the human race will only incur the wrath of their very human natures and hasten our lesson. Continuing to believe ourselves above the laws of nature will only increase the likelihood of mass malfunction and disease. Failure to recognize the need for a sustainable future robs us of that very future. We need to wake up before we are rudely awoken.

So where to start? Do we trust the politicians? Not while their chosen currency remains money and the popular vote. Do we trust our religious leaders? Not unless we want more wars based on which book we read. Do we, in fact, trust anyone in power? No, because power corrupts and the reason it corrupts is that it gives rise to a much more primary emotion: fear. The more power a person has, the more they fear losing it. And the tighter they hold on to this power, the more imbalance they cause.

Once we acknowledge the fact that the driving force behind any action, at any time, is only ever either fear or love, we can assess our own and other's motives much more clearly. It is the final, unequivocal acceptance of this fact that frees us from our usual position of entrenched self-protectionism and allows us to move forward. Given the chance, this better understanding will dissipate the fear which paralyses individuals, families, societies and nation-states and, in so doing, will lay the foundation for the peace which must precede global holistic health. Hiding behind easy beliefs and careless assumptions is no longer an option; at some level we know them to be false and the dualism which results is the cause of our internal disharmony and resulting decline in health.

The guiding principles for a truly healthy life are therefore as follows: firstly, respect for all nature (including ourselves) and, secondly, honesty in all things because truth is ultimately undeniable. Whilst struggling with daily battles and challenges, many feel that they already adhere to such principles but is this really the case? How often do small lies and political shenanigans corrupt our day? We may be law-abiding, but are our actions truly legitimate in the moral sense? Can we honestly say that we fully respect the rights of others when so much of our wealth is obtained at their expense?

Just as physical health is the outward expression of internal molecular harmony, so it is that our homes are the outward representation of our personal value system. The choices that are made in the creation and maintenance of a home act as a mirror reflecting the degree to which an individual honours themselves, humanity, the animal kingdom, the environment, the planet and the cosmos. The home is the physical conduit through which an individual connects with the world at large, not just outside their own four walls but beyond borders and across continents. Only by re-evaluating this connection can we begin to heal the rift which has opened like a chasm in humankind's soul.

In a society that encourages us to trust only that which can be seen, this connection is often obscured but, in reality, this interdependence is the mortar which binds our global home together. It is the ultimate source of holistic good health and it is up to us, the individual inhabitants of our global home, to take what opportunities we can to ensure that it is both honoured and reinforced.

Section 3

THE SPIRITUAL
HOME

CHAPTER 18

Active Healing

The ultimate arena of human existence is one of spirit and once again, our homes have a crucial role to play in enhancing our connection to this, the highest level of our being. This sense of spirit has been referred to ever since humankind began to document its own evolution. Across cultures and down through the centuries, humankind has alluded to the knowledge that there is far more to the human experience than merely eating and breathing and, whilst different names and incarnations have been attributed to this elusive presence, its essence remains the same. Prana, Chi, God-spark, consciousness: this life-force may be untouchable and uncontainable but it is never unknowable. Flowing through all things organic and inorganic, this stream of life connects us to each other, to Nature, to Earth and to the Cosmos. We are all a product of the same, original explosive event, all traceable to the same source. It is the very essence of our nature to be connected and the contentment which comes from nurturing this, our spiritual bond, is the best ensurer for health there is.

Sadly, before beginning to explore the ways in which this connection finds its expression within the home, it is first necessary to put distance between true spirit and the human-shaped power games of the religious. Early people may have needed this belief in the gods to rationalize some of the more terrifying aspects of life on Earth, but the fear that fuelled this belief was quickly seized upon as a means of gaining power, used by the few to intimidate and subjugate the many. From the Spanish Inquisition to the caste system of Hindu India, some of the most horrifying acts of inhumanity have been carried out in the name of the gods, whilst actually being in the very human pursuit of power: over people, over territory and over resources. In seeking to exploit or terrorize, aggressors frequently use the excuse of religion to defend their place on the moral high-ground, citing a 'God given right to defend ourselves' or justifying war with the pre-fix 'Holy'. But these wars are not about God or goodness: they are about control, either the flexing muscles of a greedy and arrogant nation or the desperate backlash of a dis-empowered or slighted people. By coming between the person and their essential humanity, religion has been used to blunt our innate conscience and to sanction acts of pure hate.

As thinking beings, we do not in fact need a book, a preacher or a theology to tell us what is right or wrong. If we can be truly honest with ourselves, we can each discover the right course of action or reaction to any given stimulus simply by listening to the feeling that each possible option elicits within us.

Call it conscience, intuition, a gut feeling or moral imperative this inner guidance system is always present, releasing feelings of comfort to signal the right option or feelings of discomfort to indicate the wrong. These intuitive messages are sometimes hard to hear above the din of self-delusion but choosing not to act upon this instinctive advice is what creates the conflict within us. Our ability to discern accurately what these signposts are telling us is, to a large extent, dependent on the amount of turmoil already present in our lives. How much turmoil depends on our experience of life from the moment we are born.

The young of all animals are born into the world armed with innate knowledge of how best to ensure their immediate survival. For the turtle, for instance, this means heading straight from the beach to the sea the moment they hatch. For many others, including children, it involves clamouring for parental attention. Baby birds in the nest throw their heads back and squawk loudly in a never-ending plea for the next titbit. When your dog greets you as you return home, jumping up, trying to lick your face, be aware that, as far as the dog is concerned, this is less about giving mummy kisses than about trying to get her to regurgitate her latest kill. It's how Fido gets to eat in the wild.

The more highly-evolved the species, the more complex its needs become, going beyond the physical requirements of food and warmth to include the emotional and spiritual sustenance that comes from being part of a wider social group. This pack behaviour originated in our tribal ancestry and is still evident throughout all human societies. As soon as a child leaves the family enclave and begins to socialize in the wider community, he or she becomes embroiled in playground tactics, where sub-clans are formed which exclude some whilst giving a protective identity to those accepted into the group. Whether looking at a troupe of monkeys or a group of children at play, it is soon apparent that there are leaders, followers, organizers, teachers, doers, thinkers, the brave and the caring all of whom have something positive to contribute to the group dynamic. For humans, this sense of belonging and our readiness to nurture it has been as much a contributor to our evolutionary success as has our ability to speak, for the pack mentality that still directs so much of our behaviour is the point at which our physical and emotional beings meet. Our need to be an integral part of a greater whole is an outward expression of the way in which our physical bodies have evolved. We can no more act independently of one another than can our hearts work independently of our lungs; only by acknowledging this emotional pre-requisite can happiness and physical good health follow.

As children grow, they actively seek out new clans to which they can belong: through music, fashion, religion, sport or politics. Even in adulthood, the need to be included in the group, to be respected by our peers and sure of our place in society, continues unabashed. Today, despite all our apparent sophistication, failure to acknowledge this pack mentality as an inherent part of our psyches still causes us to run into major problems as individuals. When we lose sight of our need to belong to the pack, to be a valued part of it and to have a clear role within it, all sorts of problems begin.

Unfortunately, it is all too easy to slip into a lifestyle which alienates us from each other. The apparent freedoms of the modern age have increased the likelihood of families living at great distances from one another, whilst work patterns have shifted from 9-to-5 to 24/7, taking an inevitable toll on family life. For too long, the adult desire to have all options available at all times has taken precedence over the socialization of our young. The effects have been little short of catastrophic.

For a child to be successful in terms of their relationships and life's work, they require *proactive* as opposed to *reactive* parental (along with other significant adults') interest: i.e they need attention that is given lovingly and spontaneously before it is demanded. Unfortunately, many human parents make the classic mistake of happily ignoring good behaviour and only attending to what is deemed bad. But it should be remembered that attracting parental attention is a biologically-programmed survival technique and not a behavioural choice; if the only behaviour rewarded with attention is bad behaviour, this is what will be repeated as this is what the child sees as being successful.

Meanwhile, the behaviour of the adults who are significant to the child teaches them the values of honesty, integrity and compassion. Any hypocrisy in this area, whether from parents or society, will lead to mistrust and the lack of a reliable framework of reference from which the child can find guidance. Children who are brought up in a harmonious home, nurtured from a place of love and shown demonstrably just and consistent codes of behaviour, will be secure in their place in the family and so happy in themselves. They will quickly recognize and assimilate patterns of positive reward, creating a cycle of good behaviour and congenial relationships which the child soon learns to prize over disruption. When parents and society both begin with the assumption that the child is inherently worthy, s/he will act to meet that expectation in order to maintain the harmonious energy of the pack. A child who learns the habits of openness, understanding and love will then attract similar energy into their field. On the other hand, if the prevailing pack energy is one of chaos or aggression, the child will learn to reflect or refract that energy and the disorder and disharmony will be affirmed and continued.

Any child who is routinely ignored or left alone will become insecure, frightened and desperate to find a way back into the family fold. It is then that they begin to employ ever more aggressive behaviour in order to elicit the desperately-craved parental attention. If this attention continues to be denied, the loss of place they feel leaves them in an emotional and spiritual vacuum. As overwhelming despair, anger, bitterness, and even hatred floods in to fill the void, strength is sapped and eventually the child seeks a new pack, any pack, because belonging is necessary for survival. When emotionally-immature children are forced outside of the home to find a new, more readily embracing family, they are vulnerable to all sorts of unhealthy influences, for they do not yet possess the energetic strength, or self-confidence, to resist what they may instinctively know to be wrong. This new family creates and strengthens its identity through non-conformist behaviour, happy to place itself outside of the society by which it feels collectively spurned. It is here that youth gets its reputation for anti-social behaviour and society responds by repeating the original parental mistake of refusing to acknowledge the legitimate needs of these children, focusing solely on the need to punish what it perceives as disruptive behaviour. The sub-clan now finds itself further excluded from the benefits offered to those who have stayed within the mainstream and has no choice but to become fully illegitimate in order to survive both emotionally and physically.

Even in homes where two motivated and loving parents are present, the needs of the child can become secondary to the pressures of work and the perceived need to maintain the chosen lifestyle. If adults are too tired or stressed-out to share in the lives of their families, then family members, including adults, will simply turn outside the home in order to get those needs met. This gradual process of estrangement further alienates one from the other, resulting in the eventual dissipation of the family. The key to preventing this spiralling process of alienation is inclusion, both within the home and in society; only when the much sought-after parental energy embraces all of society's children will a more cohesive future manifest.

While instilling positive values in children is an adult responsibility, grown-ups are left to take responsibility for themselves. Society strives to underline its expectations regarding our behaviour by inflicting strict laws with predictable consequences for any contravention. The vast majority of people respond by acquiescing to these rules, preferring the harmonizing energy of law abidance to the disruption and stress of life outside these imposed boundaries. However, there is a small proportion of people who have neither internal, moral policing nor any regard for society's rule of law. When this is the case, individuals are said to be sociopathic, i.e. they routinely exhibit behaviour that contravenes the moral framework of their particular society. They ignore the rights and values of others, feel no guilt and are seemingly impervious to punishment. The callousness, aggression, hostility and irresponsibility displayed comes from an emotional immaturity which shows that such people have little care or understanding of the impact of their actions. However, as is being witnessed right now, societies, governments and big business are equally capable of behaving in such a self-serving way, giving little or no thought to the peoples they are hurting. In both our own country and on the world stage, those who govern are initiating systems of practice which contravene the basic moral and social codes that allow human society to operate in harmony. The result is all too predictable.

The parent/child relationship that has been carefully nurtured and sustained in the international arena carries with it the energy of aggression and suppression. For in this analogy, the self-appointed parents are the ones with economic power (i.e. the nations of western Europe and, more recently, the US and Japan) and their unwilling children the ones without. This power was achieved through the exploitation of the resources of the New World and has been retained by forcing a system of trade rules, trade-offs and puppeteering which has left many resource-rich countries beholden and bankrupt. In their *loco-parentis* role, wealthy countries condescend to offer their charity whilst ensuring that the weak stay weak through the strong-arm tactics of institutions such as the World Trade Organization, the World Bank and the International Monetary Fund. Added to this injustice is the fact that these self-appointed parents set themselves up as leaders, guardians and protectors, thereby assuming a kind of moral, social and economic self-righteousness guaranteed to offend and irritate everyone else. The hypocritical nature of this arrangement is becoming increasingly transparent to all those concerned, as the dictatorial parents inevitably reveal themselves to be nothing more than bullies. Once the mantle of superiority slips, the disillusionment and anger of those deceived or coerced bubbles up and rightly so. For as long as the legitimate rights of these 'children' are ignored, it can come as no surprise when one or two of the more wilful ones go outside the imposed boundaries in order to survive.

If individuals, groups, societies or nations are denied their rightful place in the pack, if they are excluded from operating legitimately within the familial, societal or global fold, then alienation, separation and ultimately confrontation will follow. Until we in the West are ready to own up to the gross injustice and exploitation that is integral to the maintenance of much of the lifestyle we have come to expect, we must also be ready to accept the anger of those we abuse. For too long we have focused on our own short-term wants and needs without questioning the long-term cost. Only by recognizing that the gains which we have enjoyed are unsustainable and ultimately destructive to our planet and its people can we begin the process of redress. We have an imperative, both as individuals and as societies, to take responsibility for our actions and act truthfully, and that means morally and ethically. Failure to do so brings the kind of global disharmony that leads to war, terrorism, civil unrest, poverty, disease and environmental destruction. By ignoring the fact of our inherent, spiritual connection we absolve ourselves of our responsibility to all that forms our planetary ecosystem. In doing so, we fail ourselves, our fellow human beings and the world which we are privileged enough to share.

This next section is therefore concerned with the role of the home in moral and ethical growth. By reassessing the interaction that goes on between ourselves as family members and with those we see as outsiders (i.e. our neighbours, friends and the wider local and global community), the home is seen as a primary motivator of the spirit of family life. When the choices that are made inside our four walls are evaluated within a global context, we become more aware of the impact and repercussions of those choices. Developing this awareness can present a real challenge as it frequently causes us to question some of our most long-held assumptions and easy beliefs. But doing so means that we can begin to make the kind of informed choices that will eventually bring ourselves and our global home to the place of justice, equality and sustainability that is so necessary for the survival of ourselves and of our species.

CHAPTER 19

Family and Friends

Not only should the home provide the individual with a place in which to rest and re-fuel, it should also form a loving embrace that encompasses the entire family group. The home and the life which it encapsulates forms the framework through which all other experiences are filtered; such is the impact of its influence that its role needs to be positively enhanced wherever possible. The aim is to create a home which actively encourages inclusion, one which respects each member of the household and engages them in family life. In this respect, the concern is not so much with design or furnishings but with atmosphere: the subtle message encoded in the walls of our very own protectorate state.

The family is a dynamic unit, constantly shifting in terms of both size and need. By becoming aware of the family's changing requirements, the home can be re-interpreted on an ongoing basis in order to ensure that all those needs are met. As the family grows, it may be that the original designation of rooms needs to be re-thought. One of the greatest gifts that you can give your children is the time and space for child-led play i.e. play which is not adult directed and not intrusively supervised: just playtime with peers, secure in the knowledge that the adults are within calling distance if needed. It is this type of play that allows children to develop all the skills required for social maturity: team playing, negotiation, consideration for others, consequences, self-respect, leadership skills and so on. Setting aside space within the home for this to happen is a valuable investment and, if bedrooms are a bit small, it may be more appropriate to have the room which was originally designated as a dining room become a playroom or den. This way, your children and their friends have somewhere safe to play games, talk, listen to their music, watch television or videos of their choice and just hang out, away from parental eyes and ears but still within the family fold. Family meals and special occasions can still be accommodated even if the table is folded down when not in use. As an alternative, the adults could choose to relinquish the sitting room on those occasions when their children's friends come around and could extend the use of another room instead to include a quiet area for reading and hobbies.

Neither party should feel that the adult's needs have been supplanted, but it is for the parent to be aware of the child's need to have space to work out the complexities involved in growing up. This becomes especially important with the onset of the teenage years when children begin establishing their independence. Creating a den-style room shows that you value their need for space, whilst maintaining a family focus and so avoiding the scenario of everyone disappearing out of the door as soon as possible. The key is to be flexible with regard to the changing needs of the family and to remember that you can always reclaim all of your rooms once they've flown the nest.

Having decided on room use, remember the different energies of each colour hue. To encourage communal gathering in the shared rooms of the house, choose the warming tones of red, orange and yellow, with their implicit invitation to share ideas, feelings and concerns. Remember that a communal room has to appeal to many personalities in many moods, so it is advisable to keep the colours earthy and grounding in nature. If you wish for more vibrant colours, choose a neutral background with a variety of stronger highlights, which will draw the eye as needed. Warmth of hue and texture will encourage the family in, whether around a table, a fire or even a central rug. See the relevant chapters for more details.

Inclusion can be further encouraged through the thoughtful placement of furniture. If you are all within each other's eye-line whilst watching television, you are far more likely to chat about what's going on than if you have to turn your head to talk. Similarly, rounded, square or oval dining tables allow for ease of eye-contact and conversation far more readily than refectory-style oblong ones. Think about the messages that your furniture sends; it should be saying, 'It's comfy here; stay and relax,' rather than the harsher, 'Get off! You're ruining my lines,' so often implied by elegant design pieces. Provision of a seat or stool in the kitchen, preferably with an accompanying table, means that a visitor, whether family or friend, is far more likely to linger and chat to the cook. By encouraging your household into the kitchen, you can foster the notion of food and mealtimes as an integral part of family life, rather than an interruption to their day that manifests from nowhere. All too often, food and mealtimes become a battlefield if each member of the family has a different social schedule; however, they must remain high on the agenda. It's better to negotiate on times that suit all than to go down the slippery slope of missed meals and making do.

As with mealtimes, negotiation is the key to success where the allocation of jobs around the house is concerned. You may be of the opinion that school is a child's work and their only responsibility but, if you need them to help, try to negotiate around what they enjoy and feel interested in. It is better to trust them to walk the dog or water the flowers, both of which would have taken time out of your day, than to engage in an endless battle to complete a job done begrudgingly. The chances are you'll only have to redo it. Most adults hate housework, so why should children be expected to do it for free and not complain? Another possible way forward is to attach a little ceremony to the event. A marathon Saturday morning cleanup becomes a frenzy of communal activity, complete with music, treats and (dare it be said?) fun. By giving children specific tasks which they can accomplish with a degree of success, they can feel pride in what they've achieved.

It's a question of emotional investment and reward and, as such, is another lesson for life.

One of the more tricky aspects of communal living, be it a multi-generational family or a group of adults, is decision-making. Recognizing and respecting the rights and wishes of all members of the household is at the heart of harmonious family life; by including everyone in the decision making process, their energy becomes engaged within the heart of the home. However, where children are concerned, it must always be remembered that it is the parents' job to take responsibility for the big picture. Making decisions can feel like a heavy burden and many well-meaning adults inadvertently overwhelm children with sheer choice. It's hard enough for an adult to think what they'd like for tea tonight but, for a child who has just spent the morning negotiating the complexities of nursery, it's a whole other stress to deal with. At any age, children will find it much less challenging to make a choice between two or three fixed alternatives rather than having to come up with an idea from scratch. That said, when it comes to choosing the décor for their bedrooms, children can be allowed real creative input. This event often comes as a result of the family's moving from one area to another and, at this time of huge upheaval, having input into the decorating of their new room will encourage children to feel grounded in this new phase of their lives. Choice of colours, style and furniture placement will tell you a lot about how your child is experiencing their world and, by allowing them to express themselves, it shows them that you value this world simply because it's theirs.

When children are fully engaged within a harmonious and loving home, they learn that they have rights and value as individuals. The self-respect and security which this knowledge engenders brings forth the emotional development necessary for recognizing that others have rights and value, too. Accompanying this growing sense of self is the realization that we do not operate solely as individuals or even as family units but are, in fact, wholly a part of and party to a wider community. The more our awareness grows, the more likely we are to peek over the proverbial fence and assess the extent of our impact on others, beginning with those with whom we share our street, our view and frequently our walls: our neighbours.

❀ ❀ From Home to Community ❀ ❀

Whilst some people are blessed with the pleasant, considerate type of neighbour, others have to endure the nuisance and misery of the selfish type. Society is now beginning to take the problem of troublesome neighbours and the devastating effects that their noise/rubbish/nocturnal habits can have more seriously but, in terms of creating our own holistic home, the first consideration is not what to do about neighbours but how to be better neighbours ourselves.

When considering neighbourly responsibilities, it is important to remember that it is a person's mental or emotional relationship to the cause of any external intrusion that predisposes their reaction to it. This alerts us to the fact that, if one neighbour is already inclined towards feeling irritated by another, almost anything that neighbour does will reaffirm that dislike. Similarly, if someone feels that they have no control or right of redress over the interference being forced on them, any discord feels as if it is being amplified in direct correlation to their mounting stress levels. There are many reasons for potential dispute between adjoining households; by being on the best possible terms with your neighbours, any out-of-the-ordinary disturbances made by either party are far more likely to be tolerated.

One of the most common causes for complaint between neighbours is noise and, whilst all new flats are supposed to have built-in noise reduction measures, many older houses and conversions lack sound insulation of any kind. This is sometimes a question of cost-cutting on the part of the developer but, more often, it is simply because these homes were built in an era that predated electronic sound systems, the myriad of electrical appliances now found in the average kitchen and the shifting patterns of work and sleep. Appliances such as stereos, televisions and computers are common to most homes today and, because of our 24-hour lifestyles, they are all busy generating noise with no guaranteed periods of respite. As far as the householder is concerned, a television may be on simply for company, in which case their brain's filtering system allows it to go virtually unheard. They have control over it, they can turn it off if it bothers them, and this makes it easy to ignore.

The same can't necessarily be said for the poor neighbour who is trying to focus on who knows what but can't because he or she is driven to distraction by the same noise that the householder is happily ignoring.

Taking the time to become objectively aware of the noise we make allows us to assess its impact on others and so to take steps towards becoming a more considerate neighbour. A good first step is to invest in a portable music system or remote speakers, rather than playing the fixed one at full

volume to reach you wherever you are in the house. Turning the volume
down a notch or two will do wonders for your neighbour's stress levels without causing a strain on your hearing. And whilst the recent trend for throw-
ing out carpets may be a good one as far as dust-mites are concerned, it is not
such good news for the poor couple downstairs who are now privy to your
every conversation and movement. So, be a thoughtful neighbour and put
down rugs or carpets with absorbent underlay along the main areas of use,
particularly walkways and stairs.

Being a good neighbour is not just about noise: it's also about space.
Keeping one's own home tidy and well-maintained represents a communal
investment in the shared area of the street, village or town and, furthermore,
works to subtly encourage others to do likewise. Become aware of how your
space may be affecting your neighbours, either by spoiling their view, intrud-
ing on their privacy or encroaching on their property. One classic complaint
arises from the inadvertent blocking out of light and the culprit is frequently
the all-too-familiar *Leylandii* tree. It never asked to be planted in our gardens
yet, such is its denseness and height, it is often the cause of much garden
rage. Dense shade can obliterate the possibilities of a garden whether you're
a Sun worshipper or not as flowers, lawns, shrubs and pot plants will all suffer from being denied their time in the Sun. The tree's owners are often
blissfully unaware of the impact they're having as they will still be basking in
sunshine. Of course it's not just *Leylandii*, all trees and tall shrubs, including
climbers and ramblers, can begin to impinge upon your neighbour's domain.
Many may welcome this softening of the lines of demarcation, but don't take
it for granted. Being downwind of a festering heap of garden waste can also
cause offence, as can overflowing household rubbish, animal faeces and rotting carpets. Even the most fastidious of gardeners can inadvertently cause
problems for an organic neighbour by spraying pesticides with abandon. No
person or house is an island and all must live and equally let live but, by keeping an objective eye on one's own behaviour and expectations, a cycle of consideration and co-operation can be initiated that brings benefits to all.

Creating a harmonious relationship with one's neighbour is a very sound
investment as an ongoing, friendly communication makes it that much easier to instigate constructive dialogue should any more complex issues arise.
Furthermore, a good neighbour can be on hand to provide practical support,
such as helping out in a crisis or the sharing of emergency tools and knowledge, without necessarily involving the emotional complexity of a friendship.
The subtle nature of the neighbourly relationship allows us to co-exist but
with clear boundaries to safeguard our mutual privacy. Sadly, we often feel
so stressed in our daily lives that we draw back from further involvement with
others. But, in fact, most people are very gifted in their ability to read situations and are generally acutely aware of the difference between friendly and

helpful as opposed to nosy and pushy. The give-and-take nature of the situation really encourages us to do as we would be done by; this serves us well, as it reminds us of our own expectations as well as our own responsibilities and shortcomings.

Taking the trouble to know your neighbours (and not just the ones next door but those over as wide an area as is feasible) is especially important where children are concerned. Your child is going to meet people anyway; just because someone is unknown to you does not mean that they are unknown to your child. The old message of never talking to strangers is actually rather unhelpful because of the speed at which those intent on harm can befriend a child. It is better to have named people and designated safe houses that children know they can go to if worried and a bit far from home. The loss of the local policeman, school buses and the unwillingness of parents to allow their children to play unsupervised in the street means that the community loses the habit of everyone looking out for each other's kids. The only hope of knowing if there is a stranger in your midst is to know the locals in the first place.

Ultimately, it is only by leaving the house and getting involved in what's going on outside one's own four walls that one can hope to build the sense of belonging that is so essential to the maintenance of community spirit. Often, a school or the church becomes the focus for a young family but, if these are not appropriate, there are plenty of other ways of getting to be a local. One of the easiest and most relevant is to ensure that you regularly use the local facilities. After all, you moved to your present home because you liked the area and, by using the shops, post office, cafes, pubs, cinema, theatre and library, you will ensure that they remain viable enterprises.

If your interests take a more particular form, find out if there is a local horticultural society, walking group or amateur dramatics society, for example, in your area. You'd be surprised what's out there. And if it's not, why not think about offering your home as a base for starting one, you could be just the person everyone's been waiting for. Many neighbourhoods have their own Associations that can act to communicate the needs of the area to the council and other agencies. If you feel that you have the time and energy, this can be a great way to get involved at a hands-on level. You may not have direct, political power but an active committee can lobby for local issues, instigate festivals, cleanup days, fundraising for local projects, area plantings as well as forging links to neighbouring communities.

Community sports teams are another great way of bringing people together. The expectations of conduct encoded in the rules and regulations that allow any sport to be played satisfactorily teach us a lot about the rewards available when one 'plays the game'. Apart from being healthy on a physical level, sport espouses the principles of team-building, loyalty, fair play and good sportsmanship; qualities which are often quite difficult to acquire outside the communal field but which are, of course, very relevant to both family and professional life.

Neighbourhood projects, local clubs and sports teams are an invaluable resource and should be encouraged by residents, community groups, schools, councillors and politicians. Too often, money and space is given over to profit-making enterprises which exclude local people (or a significant proportion of them, at least). Youth frequently has little or no money but, rather than simply picking up the bill for the resulting frustration, society should invest in young people's abundant energy and channel it towards creative enterprise. It is only by encouraging a sense of belonging that respect for the self and pride in one's home can be engendered, thereby helping to prevent some of the community degradation that occurs when people feel alienated from their home environment.

CHAPTER 21

The Market-Place

Our responsibility towards our fellow human beings far exceeds the immediate embrace of our own family or community, for we are now all inhabitants of the global village; a phrase which should remind us not only of our mutual home but also of our mutual responsibility.

Today, as trade becomes the defining characteristic of our interconnection with the rest of humankind, each product chosen in the creation of a home has not only an economic value but also a spiritual value in terms of the human, animal and environmental energy taken up in its production. Whether it comes from the supermarket or the furnishing department, every item brought into the house carries with it the resonance of all that was involved in its manufacture including the raw materials, the primary producer, the traders, the corporate policy makers and the final purchaser. Only by becoming aware of the real expenditure involved in the production of any given item can a home of true value be created.

The web of human interdependence that finds its expression through trade has been increasing in complexity ever since people first sought to travel. From the establishment of the ancient silk routes that flourished between China and Europe, right up to the intricacies of modern trading, humankind has become increasingly dependent on the movement of commodities around the world in order to ensure its own survival, to supplement home-grown produce and to increase wealth. The process by which the world moves ever closer together is known historically as globalization but, in the last few decades, the speed of this apparently inevitable progression has been greater than at any time in our history. In the last five decades, world trade has grown twelve-fold and is now estimated at over £3 trillion per year, the majority of which is controlled by private business. This huge expansion should signal increased prosperity for all those involved in the chain of production but, sadly, the modern interpretation of commerce has been manipulated by people whose primary interest is not profit but profiteering.

Behind the heady words of freedom and trade, the small print shows that while some have indeed been enjoying a bonanza others have been paying a hefty toll. Figures from the Co-operative Bank's Ethical Policy Unit[6] state that, despite the huge growth in international trading, 2002 saw as many as 1.2 billion people continuing to live on less than $1 a day, a figure unchanged in the preceding ten years. 54 countries were actually poorer than they had been fifteen years previously. It is this polarization of the economies of the strongest and weakest nations that characterizes modern globalization and sets it apart from its historical context.

This modern trend began to take shape during the 1970s and 1980s, when a New Order emerged from the corporate boardrooms of America. Their ethos was of validation through economic prosperity which, by definition, inferred that financial gain was the only meaningful measure of success. When the leaders of the powerful nations of the West touted 'trade, not aid', they used a language which seemed to promote ideals of sustainability and fair play. But the reality saw massive decreases in foreign aid programmes and a coercing of the poorer nations into taking on loans with which to pay off national debt. These loans came with nefarious strings attached, in the form of Structural Adjustment Programmes (SAPs) which required countries to slash spending on healthcare, education, welfare and infrastructure in order to service their new loan repayments. The direct result of these shenanigans is that poorer countries have ended up paying far more in debt interest to the banks, corporations and financial institutions of the richest countries than they have ever received in aid. The instruments of this New Order were the International Monetary Fund (IMF), the World Bank and the World Trade Organization (WTO).

These un-elected, undemocratic institutions which are dominated by the US and, to a lesser extent, Europe and Japan have become the most powerful enforcers of socio-economic policy-making our world has ever known. Whilst proclaiming the benefits of free trade through investment and movement of capital, these organizations have brought huge pressure to bear on poorer nations, compelling them to swap tried and tested, small-scale farming practices for the promised big bucks of cash-crop economies. This has frequently involved usurping farmers from land which they had worked for generations and allowing a diverse agricultural base to be replaced by monoculture. Whilst the pro-globalizers in their offices in the U.S., London and Switzerland have continued to spout dubious statistics to show benefits for all, the reality experienced by the poorer countries themselves has been somewhat different. Having been forced to follow the Structural Adjustment Programmes, one economy after another has found that the price of the cash-crop upon which they are now dependent has started to fall.

Having opened themselves up to the 'liberalization' of trade as dictated by the IMF, the WTO and the World Bank, these developing countries suddenly became prey to exploitative trade agreements and artificially low export prices for their goods, leaving a wake of financial instability, impoverished peoples and a collapsing infrastructure. All this at a time when wealthy nations have continued to protect their own agribusinesses with huge subsidies and major import tariffs. Figures from Oxfam's *Rigged Rules and Double Standards*[7] report (2002) shows that, when developing countries export to rich countries, they face tariffs that are four times higher than those encountered by the rich countries themselves. In effect, this means that for every dollar given in aid, poorer countries lose two dollars because of the trade barriers instigated against them by the rich.

The 'do as we say, not as we do' attitude of the U.S. and Western Europe is causing widespread unrest in those countries unlucky enough to have suffered the interference of the WTO, the IMF and the World Bank. In 2003, the World Development Movement (WDM) released their *Treacherous Conditions*[8] report which stated that 'over the past three years WDM has documented 238 separate incidents of civil unrest involving millions of people across 34 countries' all opposed to IMF and World Bank-imposed economic policies. What appeared as an invitation to the world market masked the fact that it was the poorer countries themselves who were effectively being put up for sale.

Ultimately, the reason that all this occurs is us: the consumers. If we did not buy said commodities, the whole chain from the producers through to the traders who buy and sell on the futures market and all the people in the middle would collapse. But trade has flourished for thousands of years and, of course, we do want these products, we expect to be able to get these products and, for the most part, we as individuals are happy to pay a fair price. But how can we safeguard against being party to the monstrous abuses effected by the power-mongers of Washington, New York, London and Geneva? How can we get back to a system of trade which ensures that everyone involved in the chain of production is adequately and fairly rewarded?

Before answering these questions, it is first necessary to become aware of the hidden and very human costs behind many of the staples such as chocolate, coffee and textiles which we, in this country, take for granted. These are costs which are carefully hidden by a trading system that engineers convoluted paper-trails in order to put distance between the product and the often inhumane method of production. It is here that we enter the murky world of modern slavery, the malign facilitator behind much of the merchandise offered to our insatiable consumer society. When we think of slavery, we imagine the world as it was in the 17th and 18th centuries, a world that allowed around 20 million Africans to be abducted and transported across the oceans to be enslaved in the agricultural factories of North and South America. The imperialistic greed of Western Europe saw vast profits being made out of this lethal trade and it wasn't until 1833 that the British Empire finally outlawed the practice. The end of the American civil war in 1865 saw the abolition of slavery here too and the world collectively believed that this shameful trade had once and for all been consigned to the history books.

Sadly, this has not been the case; since the Second World War, slavery has re-emerged as a flourishing anachronism within modern civilization. A massive rise in population, particularly in developing countries, encouraged people to leave their rural homelands and head for the cities in order to share in the new booming world economy. For many, this dream ended abruptly on arrival at the huge shantytowns that had mushroomed around cities such as Rio de Janeiro, Mexico City and Kolkata. These new urban sprawls had no infrastructure, no prospect of employment, nowhere to grow food or keep livestock and often not even access to clean water. Poor and without registration, the people of these shantytowns were effectively forgotten by their own governments who had no hope of being able to sustain this burgeoning urban population. These people had left the relative security and sustainability of the subsistence-farming culture and found themselves in a position of extreme vulnerability: the perfect breeding ground for exploitation.

Due to the hidden nature of slavery, it is difficult to determine the true extent of the problem but the charity, Anti-slavery International, estimates that today as many as 27 million people are being denied their basic human right to liberty and a fair wage. These include men, women and children bonded into a lifetime of hard labour as security against debts that can never be re-paid. It includes women, often thousands of miles from home, tricked or trafficked into prostitution or servitude. It includes young men and women looking to support their families but instead forced to work without pay, unable to leave and in daily fear of their safety and even their lives.

The huge rise in population has led to what is effectively a glut in the human commodity, making the modern-day slave-worker utterly dispensable and easy to replace. For the enslaved person, this translates as an often short-term relationship, based on the threat and frequent infliction of terrible brutality if they do not toe the line. Anti-slavery coalitions believe that enslavement occurs in almost every country in the world, even in those who insist that it does not. There are documented cases of individuals tricked or coerced into slavery (either as domestic slaves, prostitutes or forced labour) in countries that include Britain and the U.S. So how can this happen when slavery is outlawed in every country in the world? Once again, money is at the root of the problem. Although many law enforcement agencies endeavour to prevent such practices from occurring at a local level, decisions made at the highest level ensure that they continue elsewhere. For it is the global market that is the driving force behind 21st century slavery, as it mutates to become ever less ethical, ever less accountable and ever more greedy.

For many years, the production quotas of basic commodities such as cocoa, coffee and sugar were negotiated and regulated by international federations. This allowed the individual farmer a degree of security in knowing what his crop would be worth come harvest, thereby allowing him to invest in his future and employ his workers on a long-term and fair basis.

Unfortunately, the instigation of new trade rules prevented governments from buying their own country's produce at a fixed price, instead forcing farmers to deal with foreign traders direct. This has led to plummeting prices, further compromised by the fact that, following directives from the IMF and World Bank, so many countries are now producing the same few commodities as cash-crops that the market is flooded. As small-scale farming collapsed to be replaced by the large-scale, plantation-style estates suited to the new cash-crop economy, the poor and the dispossessed frequently fell victim to promises of work that, in reality, meant enslavement.

Coffee is a typical example of a once economically sweet market turned sour by the politics of 'free trade'. As the second most traded commodity after oil, coffee cultivation once provided an income for up to 25 million farmers with quotas monitored and prices negotiated by the International Coffee Organization. This system worked well until it was decided that the practice no longer fitted with the new vision of free trade. The original agreement on coffee quotas and prices was suspended and, almost immediately, coffee prices began to plummet. Farmers were assured that market forces would soon even out the balance and that there would be a return to more viable prices. But, of course, this has not happened. Not only have coffee prices to the primary producer remained consistently low, falling by as much as 70% since 1997, but with ever more countries following the cash-crop economy, the market is now flooded with inferior beans sold at ever-cheaper prices to an increasingly undiscerning market.

Our high-streets are now full of coffee shops thanks to the import of American television shows, such as *Ellen* and *Friends*, which helped to make the coffee bar the new place to hang out. Yet the vast proportion of the money you shell out for your coffee goes to the retailer or the roaster. By taking advantage of low commodity prices and the present consumer obsession with fashion, coffee houses are able to exploit both primary producers and consumers. When fair-trade coffee is available, it is generally offered only as a speciality choice or as an occasional 'coffee of the day'. Producers do not need the condescending gestures of such retailers: they simply require a fair price in exchange for their hard-achieved products. Surely 'exchange' is the definition of trade; otherwise it becomes simply theft.

Another cynical manipulation of the notion of free trade has come in the form of bio-piracy. This is where powerful corporations are actually attempting to register patents on staple food-crops such as rice, wheat, maize, beans and sorghum. They are taking ordinary plants which have been farmed for centuries and patenting them as if they were new discoveries. In a normal world, this would be so obviously unfair that it would be unthinkable, but the world is no longer normal or fair.

Two stories disclosed by the charity ActionAid in their *Crops and Robbers*[9] report (2001) shed light on such duplicitous dealings and expose the truly insidious nature of what now passes for free trade.

The first involves the case of the Mexican farmers who, for many generations, have been happily growing yellow beans, not only to eat but also to export to the U.S. in order to make their living. Until, that is, the president of the Colorado-based seed company, Pod-Ners, visited Mexico, took some yellow bean seeds (from whom and with whose permission is not known), grew them in his greenhouse and applied for an exclusive monopoly patent on the resulting beans. Having been granted this patent in 1999, no one else could grow yellow beans in the U.S. or import them without paying his company a royalty fee. The farmers in Mexico who had been legitimately exporting their crop for years were suddenly obliged to pay Pod-Ners 15 cents per kilo in royalties. This resulted in many already poor farmers being pushed into dire economic hardship.

In India, another American company (called Rice Tec Inc) attempted a similar trick when they sought to steal away knowledge accumulated by generations of Basmati rice growers in the Himalayas. For centuries, the local farmers have been carefully selecting and maintaining rice lines in order to ensure the continuing high quality of their produce. In 1997, Rice Tec Inc was granted a patent on all novel lines, plants, seeds and grains and their progeny in the U.S. This patent would have prohibited free export to the U.S. as well as to anywhere in the Western Hemisphere. Supported by 90 international campaign organizations, including ActionAid, the Indian government was able to mount a mainly successful campaign to safeguard what had been free to its people in the first place.

This insanity was allowed to happen specifically because of an arrangement forged by the World Trade Organization, known as the Trade Related Aspects of Intellectual Property Rights ('TRIP's') Agreement. Figures from Oxfam's 2003 report, *Mugged* [10], state that increased patent protection will cost developing countries $40 billion per year: money which could otherwise be spent on healthcare, education and welfare. That the rich nations of the West allow this daylight robbery to happen in the first place is perverse and deplorable: that already struggling nations should be forced to pay to defend their basic rights is an undeniable indictment of this new capitalist model.

Of course, it's not only food production that has been warped by unfair trade rules: the textile industry has also been sullied. In recent years, the south Asian carpet industry has come under increasing scrutiny by outside agencies interested in human rights abuses. Illegal use of child labour means that many thousands of children are locked away in dark hovels working as many as 18 hours a day in atrocious conditions, frequently isolated even from their fellow captives. Underfed and in fear of their 'masters', these children will often have been abducted or taken from their homes as collateral against loans that can never be repaid. Some are lucky enough to be rescued by teams dedicated to eliminating child servitude but it can take a lifetime to rehabilitate these trauma-scarred children and, for every child brought to a place of safety, there are unknown thousands still living each day in fear and hunger.

In the U.K., the manufacturing base has collapsed as more and more makers of products once made in Britain take their factories halfway round the world in order to exploit cheap, non-union labour and virtually non-existent health and safety codes. As manufacturing bases continue to move to ever more desperate population centres, not only is unemployment and poverty left in their wake but the cycle of destitution, exploitation and suffering continues unchecked, with no-one benefiting except shareholders and executives.

So what can we do about this rampant abuse and searing inequality? Do we join the protestors? Do we lobby our governments? Yes, by all means, but probably the most effective weapon in our armament is money: the stuff corporate business understands and the reason for the whole mess in the first place. The choices we make about which products we bring into our homes delivers the clearest statement possible straight to the stock markets of Wall Street and London. It hits traders, shareholders, policy-makers and governments. It is a powerful punch which, if aimed judiciously, will get the message across that consumers say 'yes' to trade, but 'no' to exploitation. Making such informed choices can be confusing, as many brand names aim to reassure the increasingly sceptical public with claims of rigorous internal monitoring. Unfortunately, covert investigations have shown that the promises made by these companies do not always reflect the reality as experienced by the workers in their fields and factories. Only when consumers demonstrate awareness of these issues and pressurize retailers through the boycotting of unfairly- and exploitatively-traded products can a real difference be made to the lives of millions of our fellow men and women.

As far as food is concerned, it is the FAIRTRADE mark, as awarded by the Fairtrade Foundation, that offers the public the most easily recognizable and fully independent guarantee. The Fairtrade Foundation works internationally to improve the lot of over 4.5 million people, including farmers, landless labourers and their families. They insist on the rights of all individuals to fair pay, freedom of association, access to decent housing, education and healthcare, and the ability to invest in their future. Whether it's on behalf of workers on plantations and in factories or a co-operative of smallholders, the Fairtrade Foundation gives both industry and consumers the opportunity to participate in a fairer model of trade, one that includes paying farmers and producers a fair price for their produce. It is not about charity: it is about fairness. If traders are to receive the FAIRTRADE mark, they must comply with stringent standards. These include not only the rights of workers now, but also measures to allow them to plan for the future in a world of fluctuating markets, erratic weather patterns and occasionally failing harvests. By encouraging long-term planning and stability, FAIRTRADE also endeavours to encourage environmental sustainability.

There are now over 600 different FAIRTRADE products available to the consumer, including coffee, chocolate, muesli, flowers, tea, sugar, honey, biscuits, cake, fresh fruit and juices and even footballs: all competitively-priced, of excellent quality and available in supermarkets, local shops, through mail order companies and via the internet. But it's up to us to buy them and although, at present, fairly-traded products account for less than one percent of the total food market in Britain, the signs are encouraging. Between the years 1998 and 2004, sales of Fairtrade products rose from £16.7 million to £140 million, with Fairtrade roast and ground coffee accounting for 15% of 2002 sales. If these products were not up to the standard of their competitors', they would simply not survive in such a consumer-led market.

As a further means of ensuring the health and wellbeing of food growers, support the move towards organic farming. The health risks involved in long-term exposure to chemical pesticides, herbicides, fungicides and fertilizers includes organ and nerve damage, immune system impairment, breathing difficulties and hormonal disruption. By investing in organic food, the householder can encourage the move away from the intensive farming methods that do so much damage, not just to the environment but also to farming communities both at home and abroad.

Meanwhile, in India, Pakistan and Nepal, the carpet industry is being monitored by a scheme named 'RUGMARK', which exists in order to independently inspect and license loom workshops. In order to earn the RUGMARK endorsement, carpet makers must meet strict stipulations, guaranteeing that no worker is under the age of 14 years and that all workers are paid at least the minimum adult wage. Furthermore, they must allow unannounced inspections at any time. Exporters and importers pay a small contribution towards the costs involved in raising awareness and in RUGMARK's social welfare activities, which include schools, vocational training, healthcare projects and rehabilitation centres not just for the many thousands of rescued children but also for their families and their communities. Since their beginnings in 1994, RUGMARK has helped to establish primary schools, day-care centres and awareness programmes and, thanks to the commitment of traders and retailers, has effected a huge shift in the attitudes that once allowed many thousands of children to suffer the misery of hazardous and exploitative work. By 2002, almost one fifth of all Indian rugs sold in the U.K. carried the RUGMARK label while 65% of Nepal's carpet industry is now registered with them. This is wonderful progress, yet many high-street retailers still continue to stock

Indian, Nepalese and Pakistani carpets and rugs which do not carry the RUGMARK endorsement. Many claim that they have their own code of practice yet, without objective, outside scrutiny, these are hardly reliable. On the other hand, if we, the consumer, demand the RUGMARK endorsement, we can rest assured that the rug which adorns our home will not have been made by a terrified and exploited child.

Many high-profile companies are finding it increasingly hard to square their well-publicized ethical failings with their newly-informed and increasingly-politicized customer base. Continued pressure by charities, action groups and consumers has led several high-profile companies to take steps towards becoming more ethical both in their treatment of their workers and the environment. But the fact that they have had to be shamed into doing so is deeply depressing. It means that, rather than trusting in fair political and economic policy-making, consumers have to seek out information for themselves in order to decide which products conform to ethical codes of production. With time and continued pressure, this may change and we will once again go back to the days of paying a fair price for a fair deal, knowing that the monies made will benefit all those involved in the chain of production. How quickly this change comes about depends on how fully we embrace our power as consumers. Only by putting our money where our mouths are can we hasten this process and one of the most direct ways is through our own personal finances.

In the U.K., the Co-operative Bank is the only high-street bank with an independently-audited ethical investment policy. This policy is based on customer consultation and has resulted in a very transparent set of promises as to what they will and will not invest your money in. Strict criteria have to be met in terms of human rights issues, animal welfare and ecological impact, allowing the customer the peace of mind of knowing that their money is not being used to aid oppressive regimes, abuse human rights or cause ecological devastation. Ask your bank if they have an ethical policy and see what they say.

By waking up to the power in our pockets and making a commitment to buy into only those products and businesses known to be free of the taint of misery and coercion, we will be able to hasten the change to truly fair trade. Doing so will not only bring an immediate improvement in the lot of many, it will begin to strengthen the bonds of humanity, long weakened by the clawing degradation of exploitation.

But it is not only humankind we have to think about: the environment is suffering, too. As natural resources are similarly plundered, the danger is that we are creating areas which will soon no longer be able to support human life. Therefore, the role of the home in environmental degradation is to be looked at next.

CHAPTER 22

❀ ❀ ❀   Our Global Home   ❀ ❀ ❀

Astronomers tell us that everything contained within the universe is the result of The Big Bang, a momentous explosion that occurred anything up to 20 billion years ago and away from which we are all still journeying. Within this universe there are a dizzying array of phenomena: constellations, galaxies, black holes, meteors, comets, planets, stars, dark matter, supernovas, quasars, pulsars. But as far as is known, there is only one life-supporting entity, our beautiful planet home: Earth. As the universe cooled and expanded, a serendipitous meeting of electrons, protons and helium nuclei resulted in the formation of atoms, which were the prelude to all that has formed and continues to form life on Earth. We are all here as a result of that first combustion, yet never have we been so alienated from our world or from those with whom we share it.

The arrogance that characterizes our present worldview has led us to believe that we are beyond the cosmic forces that spawned us. From behind the barricades of our manmade fortresses, the human race seems unaware of the precariousness of its situation, collectively believing itself to be well-insulated against the fickleness of the elements and supported by an invulnerable biosphere. In fact, such is the inconsistency of human behaviour that, whilst happily spending thousands of pounds investing in our individual futures through the upgrading of our homes, we simultaneously invest in our collective downfall through our wilful sabotaging of the environment. If we could spend less time focusing on the aggrandizement of our private houses and more time investing in our relationship with our global home, we might yet be able to create an endowment worth having.

In the last few hundred years, the nature of our relationship with the Earth has changed dramatically. The word 'landscape' gives us a clue to our changing perceptions; in comparison to humankind's long residence on the planet, it is a concept which dates back only a moment yet it implies a distancing of ourselves from the natural world. For a long time, our surroundings were simply the world in which we lived; we did not sit back and objectify them as an artist would in a painting or a designer would in a garden. Cottages built during the 17th, 18th and 19th centuries rarely face what would now be termed the view, instead taking their orientation from the need for shelter from prevailing winds and access to natural light.

Humankind may have been cultivating and manipulating its natural environment on a small scale for thousands of years, but it was the industrial revolution that suddenly put distance between the pastoral practices of our predecessors and the new reliance on industry and technology.

As our environs became more urbanized, the naturalness of the country-side suddenly came into focus as an entity distinct from ourselves; soon, the great landscapers of the 18th and 19th centuries began adapting and simulating the natural environment to form gardens and parkland for the landed gentry. As Lancelot 'Capability' Brown and his friends sought to recreate the wonders of the natural world within the specified confines of a garden, we saw the beginning of a journey that would lead ultimately to every square inch of Earth being roped off and labelled. Hence we now have National Parks, Sites of Special Scientific Interest, designated areas of natural beauty and the green belts that surround our major cities. Although, for the most part, these are a good thing as they act to protect at least some of the world's resources and diversity from rampant exploitation by humans, they have managed to give the world a sort of theme-park identity, with the subtle inference that it's all put there for our fancy.

The mighty forests which once covered the Earth, supporting an abundance of life-forms and eco-systems, have suffered ever since the 14th century, when vast swathes of hardwoods were cut to build the ships required by Spain, Portugal, Holland and Britain for trade and warfare. But it is in the last one hundred years that the unprecedented rise in human population has placed the greatest strain on the planet's resources. Misguidedly, humankind has sought to feed itself by adopting a highly intensive, chemically-reliant system of farming that has led to the over-exploitation of both soil and farmed animals. Not only has our population exploded but our diet has become increasingly meat-based, meaning that the production of grain has had to rise not only to meet our own needs but also to feed the livestock which is so integral to Western-style diets. Maintaining such high yields from increasingly impoverished soil has necessitated a massive rise in the use of synthetic fertilizers and pesticides; as pests and diseases mutate, so increasing amounts of these chemicals are needed, causing the degree of toxicity to spiral.

As more and more countries are bullied into leaving behind traditional, mixed farming methods and to take on the monoculture of the cash-crop economy, humankind has sacrificed its once resilient and diverse global store-cupboard to be left instead with rotting food-mountains and degraded, exhausted soil, good for neither man nor beast. By coming to rely on fewer and fewer basic food-crops, humankind places itself in a very vulnerable position, just imagine the catastrophe we would face if one of these crops were to fall foul of a pandemic.

Sadly, humankind seems unable to heed even the direst warnings. The people of Ireland suffered a long and terrible famine when the crop upon which they relied as the basis of their diet was afflicted by potato blight. And in the 1930s, poor farming practices compounded by the onset of drought allowed unfettered winds to render the once-fertile plains between Kansas and Texas barren. Such was the extent of the ensuing erosion that the area eventually became known as the great Dust Bowl of America. But did humankind learn from these lessons? No, it did not. Similar problems are now manifesting in Africa, Russia and Australia as intensive farming practices, combined with the effects of wind and soil erosion, cause once-fertile soil to become unusable, thereby laying waste to the very land upon which we once relied to feed us. Vast tracts of forest are being ripped from the soil to meet the demand for agriculture, urban development, mining and timber, not to mention the many thousands of hectares lost to wildfires with each dry season.

Even the tropical rainforests, whose proximity to the equator spared them the ravages of the great ice ages, are now under threat. After 150 million years of being, these complex ecosystems, which are home to 50% of the world's flora and fauna, are being felled at an unprecedented rate. Humankind may never know what has been lost in terms of medicinal herbs and other natural wonders which have been scoured from the land by avaricious timber merchants and land-hungry developers. A 2001 *Forest Resources Assessment*[11] report from the UN Food and Agriculture Organization states that, between 1990 and 2000, there was a net reduction of forest estimated at 9.4 million hectares per year. That's a devastating 17.9 hectares every single minute. These are trees upon which we rely to purify our air, protect our watersheds and to stabilize the very ground upon which we walk.

Such is our naive presumption that the world will recover from our interference that, despite all the evidence of plummeting fish-reserves, many governments are still resisting the notion of limiting fishing in order to allow stocks time to regenerate. Many of the world's most commercially-important fish stocks are either being exploited at the very limits of sustainability or are in actual decline, including family favourites such as cod, mackerel and haddock. Along with pollution from agriculture, industry, desalination plants and oil-spills, over-fishing is devastating the seas that were once presumed to be so vast as to be invulnerable. Freshwater systems face similar threats worldwide; a situation which then negatively impacts on the many birds, mammals, amphibians and plant-life that depend upon those systems for survival.

Just as humankind has taken the seas for granted, so it is with the air. Ever since the latter part of the 19th century, when the process of industrialization began literally to hot up, the Earth has warmed significantly on both a regional and a global level, mainly as a result of the burning of fossil fuels. Now, as the number of livestock needed to feed the ever-growing human population increases and the rubbish left in landfill sites starts to decompose, methane levels are also rising significantly, further exacerbating the problem. The UK Meteorological Office reports that the 11 warmest years in the 144-year global instrument temperature record have occurred since 1990. Around the world the scientific consensus is that, without curbs on emissions, global temperatures will rise between 1 and 3.5 degrees celsius, with potentially catastrophic results which include the swamping of low-lying areas, storms, hurricanes and drought. Yet the vast majority of global energy needs are still being met through the burning of such fuels, further compounded by the wilful destruction of the forests: the one natural resource capable of restoring some kind of balance.

At present, only a fraction of the energy consumed by highly-developed, industrial nations is derived from renewable resources such as water, wind and Sun. And, although the development of these alternatives is beginning to be investigated, the only real solution is to begin to take serious steps towards cutting our energy consumption.

After a century in which humanity struggled with two world wars and a bleak financial depression, our very human hope was that when the good times finally came, they came to stay. In the West, the early signs of collapse seemed to go unnoticed: the polarization of wealth and power and poverty and powerlessness; the impact of climate changes on already-vulnerable regions; the twin horns of chronic malnutrition and obesity; the rise of new killer diseases and the return of some old ones. We carried on enjoying the boom years, only vaguely heeding the warnings about the ozone layer, spiralling cancer rates and disappearing species above the din of our own pleasure factory. But what masqueraded as a joyride has proved instead to be a kind of malevolent rollercoaster, a careering nightmare that could eventually derail the human race once and for all.

All manner of waste including airborne pesticides and herbicides, carbon dioxide, asbestos, radiation and any number of other toxins is being routinely expelled into the atmosphere, the oceans, landfill sites and inland waterways without the corporations and governments responsible necessarily making any kind of financial, ecological or moral redress. It is only when a disaster occurs that the public at large registers any alarm. In 1984, a toxic gas leak from the U.S. company Union Carbide poisoned nearly 300,000 people in Bhopal, India, yet the company escaped practically all liability for the loss of life, environmental destruction and continuing ill-health which resulted from its activities. The long-term, more insidious effects of these disasters are often still registering years after the responsible parties have departed, and are denied for as long as those with vested interests can get away with it. Yet it is only by taking responsibility for our actions, whether as individuals or multinational conglomerates, that we can ever hope to achieve sustainable growth. We are fast arriving at the point where the effects of our over-indulgence are going to belch right back at us; only if we are serious will we make the kind of difference necessary to improve the quality of our own lives and the future of others.

Whilst it is all very well to wave a righteous finger at big businesses and to demand more from our politicians and policy-makers, it is with us, the consumer, that the buck ultimately stops. If we insist on overheating our houses and driving our cars for every tiny journey we make, we cannot complain about a suffocating atmosphere, choked cities and flash-flooding. If we demand cheap food, we have to accept the consequences of nutritional deprivation and high levels of water, food and airborne toxicity. If we can't be bothered to ensure that our new dining-room table carries the Forest Stewardship Council label, then we really cannot bemoan the fact that there are no pretty rainforests to visit on our next adventure holiday. And, finally, if we insist on buying into artificially low-cost air travel, whose responsibility is it if we get badly sunburnt due to a lack of ozone? Put simply, we have to take onboard our own, personal accountability and begin to act as individuals.

Back at the house, each of us must look again at our habits and assumptions and decide how we feel about the outcomes. Speak to anyone under the impending threat of a neighbourhood incinerator or flight-path and they will generally let forth a stream of objections, and rightly so. But ask them how many bags of rubbish they throw out each week or the number of air-miles they feel they are entitled to travel every year and the answers may become a little more sheepish. We have to decide on a very personal level what kind of future we want and then put our actions resolutely where our mouths are.

The main area in which the individual can make a difference is firstly and most imperatively the cutting of energy consumption. Petrol, coal, gas, oil and wood: as we have seen, the impact on the environment from our use of these fuels is immense. Global government insistence and financing is needed in order to effect wholesale transition away from fossil fuels towards renewable energy sources; in the meantime, we have a responsibility to do what we can to lower our individual consumption. Households are responsible for nearly a third of all U.K. CO_2 emissions but, by making some easy-to-implement adjustments, you can significantly reduce your impact on the environment. Installing cavity wall insulation where appropriate can significantly cut household emissions of CO_2 and grants are often available to lower income households for this purpose. When replacing any appliances, invest in both your long-term finances and the environment by always making sure that the new ones carry the Energy Efficiency Recommended label and by choosing the best quality appliance you can afford.

As further steps: switch your electricity supplier to one which uses renewable sources to generate its power; turn down the heating by a few degrees; replace your old boiler with a condensing one; insulate your roof; use energy-efficient light bulbs where appropriate; use lower temperatures on the washing machine; use the washing-line or even a de-humidifier in preference to a tumble dryer; take shallower baths and shorter showers; fit thermostatic controls to individual radiators; pay attention when boiling water; have your milk delivered by the milkman, who uses re-usable bottles and drives an electric float; wear a jumper when it's cold; draw the curtains at dusk and use a hot water bottle at night. Don't just think about it, make a habit of it; not only will you cut your domestic fuel bill, you will also help to cut our global energy bill, something we are all going to have to pay in the end.

There is perhaps one lifestyle accessory above all others that has the most dramatic and visible effect on our environment: the car. As our major cities become almost gridlocked, our air choked and our atmosphere threatened, there are still some who insist on using their cars at every opportunity. Battery and even hydrogen-powered cars may be on the horizon but even they will not help to reduce the sheer volume of traffic. Instead, we should think about fuel consumption outside of the home in the same way that we have been encouraged to think about fuel consumption inside the home. Just as the notion of lowering the central heating thermostat a few degrees has been gently put to us, think about lowering the mileage done in your car. Admittedly, public transport may take a little more initial organization and the overcrowding and lateness can drive any sane person to despair but, that said, car-free travel has much to recommend it. For a start, you get to begin your day in the best possible way: with exercise. The cleaner morning air clears your head and you have the chance to breathe in the coming day. Your cardiovascular system gets up and running, your digestive system gets a chance to unwind, your muscles get warmed up and your body gets a good stretch. Getting out of bed and into a car deprives your body of this wake-up routine, so do what you know is right for both yourself and the environment and get into your stride.

One of the defining differences between geographically-removed peoples is their attitude towards water. This pre-requisite for life is, of course, cherished by those who live in countries where it is scarce and squandered by those who perceive it to be plentiful. But our world is changing more quickly than our perceptions. Population growth, particularly when it is concentrated in large urban areas, is putting huge pressure on the available water supply. According to Thames Water Utilities, the Thames region in the south east of England has less water per head of population than areas traditionally thought of as dry, such as Madrid or Istanbul. The pressure imposed by an increasing population is further compounded by lifestyle factors, which in London have resulted in a rise in individual water consumption of around 15% since the early 1980s. This amounts to more than 23 litres per person per day. The 2001 Intergovernmental Panel on Climate

Change [12] reports that 1.7 billion people (a third of the world's population)
live in regions that are water-stressed. Depending on population growth,
this could increase to nearly 5 billion by 2025. Our attitude towards water
obviously needs to be revised. In the home, there is much that can be done
to lower consumption and to preserve this increasingly precious resource.

Showers have long been touted as the economical alternative to baths,
saving on average around 400 litres of water per week. But the advent of the
power shower has closed the gap somewhat; if you're serious about conser-
vation, limit the time spent under the nozzle. Overuse of water by the toilet flush is another major source of waste. New homes are generally fitted
with eco-flush toilets, which offer two settings for your convenience; otherwise, many Water Boards offer small devices to fit into cisterns in order to
reduce the amount of water used in each flush. A homemade equivalent can
be fashioned by wrapping a large stone or brick in a plastic bag and placing
it very gently inside the cistern. A water-friendly checklist would further
include: checking your home for leaky pipes and taps; ensuring that water
appliances, such as washing machines and dishwashers, carry the Water-
Wise efficiency label and are used only when full; not overfilling the kettle
or saucepan; using a beaker rather than running water when brushing your
teeth; lagging pipes to prevent bursts in cold weather; using the cooled,
nutrient-rich water from boiling eggs (with used teabags split into it) to feed
houseplants and installing a water butt to collect rainwater from gutters for
use in the garden. Finally, ensure that all your washing is done in water-
friendly products, thereby helping to minimize the pollution that blights our
water systems. There are many readily-available products for both the home
and ourselves that are environmentally friendly, effective and reasonably
priced. But, of course, we do have to buy them if we want our homes to
cause less harm to the environment, to our families and to ourselves.

Another fundamental step to take on the road to environmental good
health is to reduce the amount of waste your household generates. Chapter
Two detailed ways in which to do this, so redouble your efforts by demanding to be deleted from irrelevant mailing lists; don't buy over-packaged
goods, but choose instead goods in low energy impact and recyclable packaging; use a reusable shopping bag rather than endless plastic bags; be honest about what you do need and what you can actually live without; get off
the up-grade rollercoaster, mending or cleaning whenever possible rather
than replacing and, if you must replace, make sure of the environmental
integrity of any new item brought into the home.

When waste is unavoidable, be responsible about its disposal. Fat
poured down drains causes huge problems for the Water Boards, as do
plumbing mistakes which can lead to water-borne household waste (such
as raw sewage and detergents) directly contaminating streams and rivers.

Further problems are caused by waste being simply fly-tipped on roadsides and on green land. Even garden waste can cause problems if the plants being dumped are rampant growers. The virulent Japanese Knot Weed was once a garden favourite but is now a rampaging pest that threatens to oust some of our native wildflowers from their traditional habitats. If you are ever in any doubt about how to discard safely, contact the council; most will have facilities for the disposal of old paint, electrical appliances, textiles and garden trimmings.

As a further step, the household can help to preserve the holistic health of our global home by following an organic, non-chemical based approach to food, home and healthcare. While switching to organic methods of food production is a very significantly first step, it is cotton cultivation that provides one of the main global markets for chemical pesticides. Organic cotton products are becoming more readily-available but more exciting still is the re-discovery of hemp as an almost miracle crop. Although traditionally prized for its ability to make strong rope, hemp is now being recognized as a true all-rounder. Not only is the seed highly nutritious, being very rich in Omega 3, 6 and 9, essential polyunsaturates and protein, but the plant can also be used in the making of clothes, shoes, cosmetics, cleaning products, paints, and even buildings. Not only is it versatile but it yields around three times as much fibre per acre as cotton plants do. Even more remarkable than this, though, is the fact that hemp is naturally resistant to insects, meaning that no pesticides are necessary for its cultivation. Hemp products are now to be found in good quality food halls, health-food shops and through specialist suppliers of all the above products. By taking a moment to explore the alternatives available, the householder can make choices which significantly reduce the demand for harmful chemicals, thereby directly reducing the harm done to ourselves and our environment and, at the same time, helping to ensure the continuing bio-diversity so essential to our future.

Just as the organic label ensures good guardianship of our soil, so other certification schemes exist to promote responsibility towards other components of our global ecosystem. The Forest Stewardship Council (FSC) provides an international certification and labelling scheme that allows consumers to identify wood and wood products that come from well-managed forests. Then there is the Marine Stewardship Council (MSC) with its distinctive blue and white fish logo that allows consumers to identify which fish and seafood comes from responsibly managed, sustainable fisheries. With many customers becoming increasingly aware of environmental issues, retailers are now recognizing the value of demonstrating responsible practice. MSC-labelled seafood is available in 24 different countries including the U.K., the U.S. and Australia, but if none of the seafood in your local supermarket or fishmongers is displaying their logo, it's up to you, the potential customer, to ask why not. It is only by using our power as consumers that we can bring our influence to bear.

You might also try to reduce the amount of meat and dairy produce eaten within your household. This would significantly benefit the environment by reducing the amount of grain needed to be grown in order to feed those animals destined for the table. Direct consumption of cereals by the human population provides a far more efficient use of land and energy resources, as a plant-based diet is cheaper and less energy-intensive to produce (as well as being healthier to eat), thereby dramatically reducing human impact on natural habitats.

Of course, humankind's ability to grow food is dependent on being able to predict the weather within reason, but weather patterns around the world are changing and even the experts can't agree on what the final outcome is going to be. Whether the end result is a drier, wetter, warmer or colder environment, what is clear is that it will put pressure on populations and the land's ability to support them. Homeowners will not be able to get insurance on land subject to repeated flooding, nor will this land be viable for farming. If Europe continues to see erratic changes in temperature, this will impact not only on the agriculture of the region but also on its carefully-nurtured tourist industry. No one wants to go on a beach holiday where it is too hot to sit on the beach or go skiing where there's no snow. As food and water shortages begin to stalk once-fertile land, people will need to seek new areas from which to find sustenance. In the past, this readiness to migrate in order to find new resources has always been an integral part of humankind's ability to survive, but never has the population been so great, nor land at such a premium. Where are we all to find new homes, new incomes and the food to sustain us in an increasingly depleted and pressurized world?

The danger is that, as this pressure builds, those in economic power will become ever more protectionist over what is left, exacerbating the process of polarization between the 'haves' and 'have nots' of the world. In reality, though, the terms of our survival may not be so easily defined. In its ongoing *Living Planet* report [13], the World Wildlife Fund uses an ecological footprint to describe the impact that we as individuals leave on the Earth. Using global hectares per head of population as a measure of our consumption of natural resources, the report estimates that the average American stomps ahead leaving a footprint of 9.5 hectares, with the British trotting behind at 5.4. Western Europeans average at approximately 5.1, while in Ethiopia and Burundi they tiptoe in at 0.7 hectares per head. This gross disparity casts shame on the economic super-powers yet, in a world under pressure, who would survive? Those made bloated and weak by years of nutritional and chemical abuse or those who know how to yield basic sustenance from an impoverished land? Is it possible that, as the resources upon which the modern world relies for its high-maintenance survival run out, the 'meek' (if you'll pardon the condescension) really shall inherit the Earth?

It is imperative that we recognize our collective responsibility for our home planet and the people, fauna and flora we share it with. Our survival depends upon it. Some signs are encouraging. Following huge investment, rivers and waterways in the U.K. are now cleaner than at any time during the last 200 years. Increasingly, grants are becoming available to encourage the installation of solar panels, draught-proofing, cavity wall and loft insulation, as well as council-sponsored doorstep collections of recycling and even low-cost compost bins. There are even some studies which suggest that the holes in the ozone layer are at last beginning to shrink. But we cannot be complacent. The fact that we can make a difference must act as an impetus to increase our efforts. As a society and as a species we cannot know what the future holds but as individuals we must recognize the need to make choices that positively influence the world as we experience it in the here and now. If we can recognize the holistic nature of our planet's functioning and put ourselves back into the equation, we will recognize that what hurts others can ultimately only hurt ourselves. Nowhere is this truth more apparent than in our relationship to and our treatment of animals.

Animal Magic

Throughout this book reference has been made to the primary need for respect for all living things. Sadly, much of what constitutes the average home will have caused distress at some level to the animal kingdom either through the decimation of natural habitats, the infliction of pain and distress by scientists in laboratories, or the horrors of intensive farming. The work of Dr Emoto demonstrated the impact of stress vibrations on a simple water crystal; this gives an indication of the detriment caused to an animal repeatedly terrified through the actions of human beings. The work of the biophysicist Fritz-Albert Popp illustrated the existence of an actual light within, a light which does not differentiate us from plants and animals but inextricably unites us with them. We know, then, that we are not single, independently-operating entities but are all part of a universal sea of energy which means that, whether one chooses to acknowledge it or not, our relationship with animals goes far beyond the need for food, beasts of burden or even companionship. For as long as these animals are suffering, we will continue to suffer too; when we inflict pain or distress on an animal, either directly or indirectly, the effect is felt at the very core level of our being. Only by waking up to the repercussions that result from its treatment of animals can humankind hope to find the answer to the only question worth asking: how do we find health and happiness?

Having already highlighted humankind's detrimental influence on the animal kingdom's natural habitats, this chapter is concerned with the direct impact that the homemaker has through their choice of food, healthcare and household products.

Despite the fact that the vegetarian diet has been shown to benefit both the environment and our health in numerous ways, our carnivorous habits seem to be so strongly ingrained in our evolutionary heritage that it is often pointless to proselytize on this issue. However, if you do eat meat or fish, it is of fundamental benefit to all concerned to eat only those creatures raised freely and compassionately and killed humanely. Once again, we must look at the farming practices that have dominated our food supply over the past few decades. As far as the poor animals are concerned, our ongoing obsession with obtaining the highest yield possible from both land and livestock has meant a shift away from the virtually free-range existence of yesteryear towards a new hell of battery sheds, pig units, farrowing crates, routine mutilation and misery. As animals have been forced to live in unsanitary, artificially-lit, overcrowded and wholly unnatural environments, force-fed an inappropriate diet and stressed into self-maiming by their terrifying new lifestyles, the utterly foreseeable has happened. They have begun to get ill.

Consider the pig. This species has spent the last several thousand years living in the forest, rooting around in the Earth, using its strong snout to snuffle out all the nutrients needed for a healthy life. Pigs live in an extended matriarchal group, with sows giving birth once a year to three or four piglets with whom the mother closely bonds. As with the young of all animals, piglets love to play and need to do so for their healthy development. The family is immensely clean in its habits and likes to roll in the mud to keep cool. The average pig is far more intelligent than the average dog, with a long memory and, as parents, quite prepared to travel up to 15 kilometres a night in search of food for their young. Having been hunted by humans for many centuries, these animals had become wary of the fate that a human could inflict. However, it is doubtful that anything could have prepared them for the impending horror they would suffer.

Pig units are one of the biggest disgraces of conventional farming. Pregnant sows are shut into barren cells, often devoid of bedding and awash with excreta, without even the space to turn around. Mothers give birth into their own faeces or are left haemorrhaging and fly-infested, unable to nuzzle their newborn piglets or to rest from them if need be. Undercover work by the animal welfare group, Viva!, has documented cases of appalling neglect, including some found on farms which supply the major supermarket chains. They have found pigs left to suffer broken legs as well as the abscesses, cuts and lacerations that result from rubbing against the restrictive metal cages in which they are forced to live. They have found animals in fear and distress, the most basic standards of hygiene ignored, disease an all-encompassing shroud. More than 90% of all piglets in the U.K. are factory-farmed: as ever, the god is profit. Why allow a pig to expend calories through natural behaviour when you can keep it in a pen so small it can hardly move? Why allow a piglet to wean naturally at 12 weeks when you can remove it at 28 days? Why worry about the diarrhoea that this causes when you can pump them with daily drugs? Why care about their immune systems, weakened by the psychological stress of their premature separation from their mothers, early weaning and by the cocktail of chemicals needed to keep them growing? OK, so they then become susceptible to diseases as devastating as E-coli, salmonella, Post-weaning Multisystemic Syndrome and greasy pig disease which can then go on to infect half the herd; who cares?

Well, *we* should, because many of the diseases afflicting these poor animals such as meningitis, pneumonia, campylobacter and salmonella are capable of crossing the species barrier and infecting humans. Furthermore, unhealthy pigs are susceptible to both human and avian flu strains, thus presenting the perfect opportunity for the strains to exchange genetic material and thereby paving the way for a global pandemic.

As the incidence of such diseases increases worldwide, the legacy of our abuse is beginning to manifest. The overcrowding, neglect and appalling diet forced on all intensively-farmed animals is taking its toll and we are now going to join them in paying the price. By routinely using antibiotics to promote growth and retard infection, farmers have been able to exploit and then sell hideously bloated and grotesquely disfigured animals and birds and still turn a profit. But antibiotic use is a non-sustainable option because of the ability of bacteria to mutate and develop resistance. Not only do the drugs enter the food-chain straight into our own bodies, but many of the bacteria from which they were originally intended to protect us have become resistant to the antibiotics presently available. The emergence of these bacterial super-bugs can be lain almost entirely at the door of avaricious farmers and complacent consumers. The insatiable demand for cheap, albeit tasteless, nutritionally-questionable meat means that it is not just antibiotics that are part and parcel of everyday intensive farming practice so are steroids, beta-blockers and tranquillizers. Fancy that in a sandwich?

The suffering endured by these creatures is appalling. The brutality of de-beaking farmed ducks, the caging of salmon, the living nightmare of farrowing crates and battery cages, live transportation across hundreds of miles all culminate in the appalling carnage of mass slaughter. Consumers often choose not to think too long or too hard about meat and fish farming, naively trusting that the government and the food industry themselves monitor farms and keep us and our food safe from any less than honourable practices. But, according to the charity Compassion In World Farming (CIWF), many of the farm-assured labels (such as the British Farm Standard or the Lion Quality mark for eggs) which have sprung up in an attempt to reassure consumers, simply mean a compliance with minimum regulatory standards [14]. Products declared farm-fresh rarely guarantee high animal welfare and are frequently just a cynical marketing tactic employed by factory farmers to confuse the unwary shopper. In 2004, the CIWF conducted an in-depth survey of ten of the U.K.'s leading supermarket's policies on animal welfare; of those they surveyed, Waitrose came top, closely followed by Marks and Spencer [15].

Ultimately, though, it is the organic Soil Association assurance that is recommended as having the highest standards of all. The only way to ensure the best quality care for the animals we eat is to buy only that produce which is clearly marked as organic. By banning the routine use of chemicals, good husbandry practices have to be relied upon to keep the animals healthy. This is good news for the animals as it requires access to open pasture, an appropriate diet and a high level of care; it's also good news for us as it means that the meat which reaches our tables is of the highest quality available. It is far healthier to eat organic meat two or three times a week than non-organic meat seven times.

With a catastrophic lack of understanding which only humans could achieve, we not only abuse, mutilate and torture the animals intended for our food we also abuse, mutilate and torture them in the name of health. Conventional wisdom (as espoused by the chemical manufacturers who dominate all aspects of our home and health) asserts that it is synthetic chemicals that keep all things well. Much of the research supporting this assertion is carried out on subjects conveniently unable to speak out about the horrific suffering that such chemicals induce. By using animals in their experiments, the chemical and biological research industry has managed to elude outside scrutiny and to remain shrouded in a cloak-and-dagger atmosphere more appropriate to MI6 than the healing profession. The reason they give for this secrecy is the distasteful nature of this so-called research, but the truth is that these industries use the passionate opposition to animal research as an excuse for keeping objective monitoring at bay. In fact, it is only this lack of external regulation that allows such a scientifically and morally-bankrupt practice to continue. In their rush to patent and market new household, pharmaceutical, agricultural and industrial formulations, chemical corporations continue to use this outmoded methodology because it facilitates their multi-billion dollar industry, whose main incentive is not health but profit.

Let's look at the facts dispassionately. Firstly (and most obviously), animals are not humans and so cannot be relied upon to tell us anything definitive about ourselves. The animals used for testing are generally selected on the grounds of cost and convenience, not on the basis of any perceived similarities to humans. Numerous products have been unleashed on the public having been deemed safe by animal testing, only to be withdrawn after adverse human reactions. Manoplax, a drug for congestive heart-failure, was tested on rats, rabbits, cats, dogs, guinea pigs, ferrets and baboons yet was withdrawn after only one year when it was found that humans taking it had a significantly increased risk of death. Zimelidine (from the Swiss pharmaceutical company, Astra) was an antidepressant whose side effects in humans included serious neurological impairment, skin disorders and death, none of which had been indicated through exhaustive testing on animals. On the other hand, aspirin causes birth defects in rats and mice but is generally safe for humans. Figures from within the industry itself admit that as many as 95% of substances passed as safe as a result of animal testing are immediately rejected in human studies. Results obtained from experimenting on animals are at best crude and at worst fatal and therefore never give a reliable indication of human responses. All in all, it is a massive waste of time, resources and, oh yes, animal lives.

The second reason that animal testing is so criminally pointless is that disease is always the culmination of many factors, including nutritional deprivation, toxicity, unresolved emotional or physical stress and, for some people, an inherited pre-disposition. Consequently, it is only by assessing all of these factors that a cure can be found. Unfortunately for the public, there is no profit in actually curing people, especially if the cure lies in naturally-occurring and therefore un-patentable remedies such as nutritious organic food, clean water, physical exercise, emotional support and the avoidance of all the afore-mentioned chemicals. Animal research into today's health headliners such as cancer, Alzheimer's, Parkinson's or diabetes accounts for vast sums of public money, both via the treasury and charities. Yet much of it is spent on inducing the outward signs of the said disease in an animal which would not (and in many cases could not) naturally get the disease itself. You simply cannot induce the characteristics of an illness and believe that you have the illness itself; it's a bit like tickling the nose of a cheese and expecting to find a cure for the common cold. The emotive chase to be The One Who Discovered the Cure for AIDS can often involve working on an entirely different virus since many species cannot be infected with HIV. In those that can, namely chimps, the virus behaves entirely differently from how it behaves in humans, just as cancer does and in fact, none go on to develop AIDS. Yet many of the major research institutions and charities still continue to fund the mutilation of animals in an attempt to induce artificial symptoms in the entirely erroneous conviction that this will tell us about the human condition. Investigation into Parkinson's Disease involves injecting toxins into the brains of marmoset monkeys; as no human falls victim to the disease through this method, the animals predictably display entirely different reactions. Furthermore, computer imaging shows that these animals' brains differ from ours so fundamentally (in terms of neural circuitry, transmission and number, location and importance of brain cells) as to render the whole exercise pointless.

This is the reality of the vivisection industry: the greatest blind alley of them all. More than any other, it is the one thing that has held back humankind's understanding of disease. Whilst every other scientific discipline and the technology which supports them have evolved at an ever-increasing rate, vivisection is back there in the Dark Ages relying on the same model for testing that it was using several hundred years ago. It's as if the industry is still tinkering with the square in the hope of creating the perfect wheel.

Frequently deprived of both natural light and an appropriate diet, and often kept in isolation, intelligent social animals (such as rats, mice, dogs, pigs and monkeys) are subjected to a relentless barrage of stress and suffering. Undercover investigations have shown food and water deprivation being used to make the animals perform certain tasks, a woeful lack of care of even post-operative animals and frequent death and mutilation resulting from poor clinical practice (let alone the death and mutilation inflicted on purpose). And, of course, it's not just drugs that require animal testing. Most high-street brands of household products and personal care items are tainted by the blood of laboratory animals. That newly scented washing up liquid: full of synthetic chemicals which are tested by being dripped into the eyes of fully conscious rabbits, animals whose tear flow is not sufficient to wash away such painful substances. That new product for getting your whites whiter: dripped onto the shaved skin of a physically-restrained animal whose skin is then monitored for redness, swelling and cracking but who is restrained from licking its wounds better. Anything from pesticides to bleaching agents may have been tested on animals in increasing doses until the lethal threshold for 50% of the trial group is reached. These notorious tests involve dripping chemical substances into the eyes of dogs, rabbits and other animals or force-feeding them either by mouth, injection or inhalation. Toxic effects include cries of pain, vomiting, tremors, convulsions, bleeding and death. After years of this barbaric practice, even scientists are condemning this test as unreliable and irrelevant. And don't be fooled by the defence of anaesthesia. By law, it only needs to be administered in order to mitigate 'unnecessary suffering'. In reality, this means that it is rarely administered, after all it all costs money.

At the end of the day, what makes animal testing so abhorrent is that it is so entirely unnecessary. Alternatives exist right now which are not only humane but to use an argument which you would imagine that commerce (not to mention people whose professed wish is to heal) heeds: reliable, cost-effective and fast. Imaging techniques, cell and tissue cultures, epidemiological studies, computer and mathematical models, artificial organs, it's all there to be taken advantage of, yet investment in these alternatives remains paltry in comparison to the millions spent annually on animal testing.

Here though, the concern is not with us humans. From the safety of our homes we can choose to eat rubbish until ill-health manifests. We can choose to bathe in chemicals toxic to our bodies just because we like the smell. We can choose to live the half-life proffered by drug dependency if we feel it's easier than changing our lifestyle. But the animals in the vivisection laboratories have no choice. They are entirely in the hands of people who wilfully and repeatedly inflict the most appalling physical and emotional pain, and who do so with money given to them by Joe and Joanna Public: through the products which they buy, through their charitable donations and through their taxes.

The brutality that goes on in these laboratories is almost too painful for the average human to face, but face it we must. Every time we buy a product that has been tested on animals, we buy into this murderous industry. It may take more than this short discourse to convince you that there is an alternative path to good physical health, but if we are ever going to rid ourselves of the fraudulent and frankly sinister chemical domination that is directly contributing to our failing health, you could begin by refusing to buy any household and personal care product that is not endorsed by the cruelty-free label.

This includes nearly all of the most commonly-available high-street brands, as well as the never-ending procession of so-called new, improved replacements for products that have been doing the job perfectly adequately for years. It also includes all the fruit, vegetables and foodstuffs sprayed with agricultural chemicals, toxic both to laboratory animals and to those in the wild. Fortunately, it is much easier to find cruelty free products these days, even in supermarkets, but beware that not all labelling is totally transparent about the methods involved. For example, 'against animal testing' does not necessarily mean that the company does not permit animal tested ingredients into its products. Of course, an ethical company could be happily using a product which another company then tests on animals. So, the best way to avoid confusion is to send off for a list of companies (and charities) endorsed by antivivisection charities, such as the British Union for the Abolition of Vivisection (contact details at the back of this book). All it then takes is a fresh look at your supermarket or a trip to the health-food store and you can once and for all remove the stain of suffering from your home.

For a proportion of people, the suffering of animals is never going to be of great importance. Humankind has always had in its midst those who enjoy cock-fighting, badger-baiting and fox-hunting, or those who think that blasting a hole in an animal who is peacefully going about its life constitutes sport in some way. But there are also many so-called animal lovers who, whilst foisting endless affection on their own pooch or moggie, continue to buy products whose ingredients have been used to inflict appalling pain and distress on animals just as intelligent and loving as their own. The saddest irony is that having a pet has been found to improve our lives immeasurably for in times of stress and sadness, it is animals who have the power to heal. A study by Dr June McNicholas, at Warwick University, looked at the effects of pet ownership on school-age children and found that it resulted in a more stable (i.e. better) immune function and was significantly associated with better rates of attendance at school. The study concluded that, providing the parents observed correct preventative regimes regarding fleas and worms (both of which can be controlled by the use of herbs rather than synthetic chemicals), the overall benefits of pet ownership far outweighed any risks.

Animals have also been used to help children with communication or self-esteem problems, as well encouraging those who have suffered from violence or drug abuse to become happier and more self-confident. This is the true magic of animals; although no one seems to know quite why, it has been proven time and again that those of us lucky enough to have them in our lives stay healthier, live longer, heal more quickly and feel happier. The Pets As Therapy charity provides a scheme where volunteers take their dogs and cats (all of whom will have been fully-vetted in terms of health and temperament) to visit those in hospitals, nursing homes, special needs schools, hospices and care centres.

The unconditional love brought by these PAT animals helps people to relax and become less withdrawn, seeming to positively influence recovery even after conditions as serious as stroke, heart attack or surgery. Dogs and horses, in particular, have served us loyally and unquestioningly in our private lives, our working lives and in our wars. Trained dogs have made huge differences in the lives of those who have lost their sight or hearing, and millions of humans have found happiness and companionship through caring for an animal. This is the true lesson we can learn from animals, that it is kindness, loyalty and friendship that are the keys to good health.

From the warmth and safety of our own homes, we must do all we can to improve the plight of the animals with whom we share our planet. Whether they are in the wild, abandoned on our streets, imprisoned in factory farms or in laboratories, it is we, at the top of the evolutionary ladder, who have a case of *noblesse oblige* of cosmic proportions. As, at last, our physicality comes into line with our spirituality, we see that when the inner light that unites all living things is dimmed in so many animals by the actions of humankind, we can only bring suffering upon ourselves. And we surely are suffering, in heart as well as in body. How much healthier and happier would we be today if we had heeded those responsibilities, set aside our arrogance and allowed animals to teach us the benefits of leading more natural, less harmful lives?

❀ ❀ ❀   The Natural Garden   ❀ ❀ ❀

Although this book is primarily concerned with the creation of a home, there follows a brief chapter on the great outdoors. Whatever the size of your patch, be it a plant pot outside the front door, a window box, a balcony or a garden, the important point to remember is that it serves to enhance your connection to nature. Plants, trees, shrubs and their attendant wildlife draw our energy out beyond the realms of our internal space and remind us of the integral part we play in the ecosystem of the planet.

Gardens have always been seen as close to godliness. The word 'paradise' is derived from the Persian word for 'walled garden' and for Muslims this precious place, watered by running streams, is the ultimate reward for a life lived honourably. In the Christian tradition, life began in the Garden of Eden, while in Japan the Shinto priests create meditative gardens in which to contemplate and connect to the beauty of nature. Early town-planners instinctively recognized the public's need for a breathing space long before the hazards of air pollution were fully understood and so created garden cities, designed with integral parks and gardens and contained by green belts of land which were protected by law against further development. As the pressure on land increases, this innate understanding of human needs is in danger of being forgotten, with cash-strapped councils and even schools selling off green space to the developers. But just as the land is becoming increasingly pressured, so are we and for many, the answer to all this modern stress is to be found in the tending of a garden.

The rewards of this gentle pastime are immense but, before we begin, a word of warning. Although farmers are regularly accused of devastating the landscape and damaging the environment through their use of pesticides, householders also cause major problems due to a lack of training in the appropriate use and disposal of these chemicals, some of which are already banned due to their hazardous nature. For not only are these chemicals toxic to pests, spores and weeds, but they are also toxic to us, causing problems for our eyes, respiratory tract, liver, kidneys and lungs. Each year, more and more chemicals are withdrawn as fears for our health and safety emerge yet sales to the householder are still booming. In 2001, the Pesticide Action Network (PAN)'s *Home and Garden Survey*[16] found that U.K. householders spent around £35 million on over 4,000 tonnes of pesticide, an increase of 78% on sales figures for 1998.

A single tablespoon of spilled pesticide concentrate is capable of polluting a day's worth of drinking water for 200,000 people, yet PAN found that 20-30% of people disposed of their unwanted pesticides by simply putting them down the drain or into the bin. And while 5-10% of people did dispose of them safely by taking them to a specialist waste facility, the most common solution of all was simply to leave the unwanted chemicals indefinitely, either in the shed or (worse still) under the kitchen sink. If you have dangerous chemicals that you want to get rid of, contact your local council or, for pesticides, see the dedicated PAN website (details at the back of the book). Better still, don't buy them in the first place. All those chemicals set up a cycle of devastation that logically can only do more harm than good. Many well-intentioned people spend all winter feeding birds with nuts and seeds, then all summer killing off their food supply with pesticides. This mania for killing off every single bug in the garden has contributed to the plummeting bird population. Once-common species such as the house sparrow and starling have seen their numbers drop by as much as 80% in just three decades, thanks to the twin pressures of reduced habitats and fewer insects to eat. If you encourage birds into your garden in the winter then you owe it to them to leave the aphids there for them to pick off come spring.

This is not a gardening book but, to get you on the right track, here is a quick introduction to some of the ways in which you can create a garden that truly grows and in so doing heals all who enjoy it.

The first decision to make before you even pick up your plant catalogue is what kind of gardener you are to be. If you are the type who is primarily interested in show: perfect blooms, manicured lawns and precision beds then you've probably stopped reading this already. This type of gardening is very artistic and, as such, interested in artifice. There is nothing neat and straight-edged about nature and the true gardener's role is more about tweaking the edges than the kind of divine intervention doled out from behind a mist of killer bug-spray. Gardens are living, holistic ecosystems, about far more than just plants and landscaping. With a little care, you can have a garden that literally teems with life: birds, butterflies, lacewings, dragonflies, frogs, toads and hedgehogs will all be drawn to a garden that provides them with their needs and does them no harm.

Secondly, you need to select plants carefully. Choose plants that are disease-resistant in the first place and then plant them where they'll be happiest, thereby optimizing their chances of flourishing without recourse to artificial chemicals. Wildflowers growing in hedgerows and meadows are not prone to the rash of weaknesses that trouble cultivated hybrids; they are inherently robust, suited to the area which they have colonized and, left untended, thrive perfectly happily for years.

If plants do need any help, nature will be able to provide it. Companion planting is a concept that has been around for so many years that much of its wisdom is known today in the form of old wives' tales and is therefore dismissed as quaint, old-fashioned nonsense by the purveyors of synthetic chemical warfare. However, agriculturists, horticulturists and gardeners have been successfully harnessing the chemistry behind companionship for years and using it as a means of naturally boosting both the health and yield of plants and their soil. One of the most useful companion plants is garlic; not only does it ward off greenfly, snails, slugs and weevils but it also enhances the fragrance of the flowers (especially roses) that it is grown alongside. (Beans, on the other hand, are not so fond of garlic; for some reason, both seem to fail in each other's company.) Try to find room in your garden for stinging nettles. Their leaves can be steeped in water for a couple of weeks to create an all-purpose feed for other plants, and they give the soil they're grown in a boost, too. Nettles also provide a place for butterflies (particularly tortoiseshells, red admirals and peacocks) to lay their eggs and, as if this weren't reason enough, you can use the youngest leaves to give yourself a natural tonic by making your own nettle tea (wear thick gloves for picking).

As we can see, using plants for their therapeutic as well as aesthetic properties shows how the natural gardener can enhance the holistic health of both the garden and the family. Plants can be used to add nutrients to the soil and deter destructive diseases and bugs, as well as boosting the inherent strength and diversity of the plot. Using robust plant species will benefit the gardener's health by avoiding the need for potentially carcinogenic chemicals and many plants can be harvested to bring their potent immune-supporting nutrients to the table. If you can only grow a few plants, either in a window box or tub, then herbs are recommended. Most are fairly unfussy but they do need to be harvested regularly in order to access their therapeutic qualities.

Herbs can be eaten fresh, steeped in hot water to make teas, infused in pure vegetable oils to create a soothing balm or applied neat to fevered skin. (Such is their potency that you should avoid excessive amounts if you are pregnant, breastfeeding or if suffering from epileptic fits and you should always get professional advice if using herbs to treat a specific illness.) Here are just a few examples of how they can be used:

PARSLEY: sprinkled fresh onto your food, this wonderful herb is full of the free-radical busting antioxidant vitamins A an C. It is also packed with vitamin B, as well as providing excellent support for the liver. As if this weren't enough, parsley also contains calcium, iron, phosphorus and potassium.

LEMON BALM: this easy to grow herb has a wonderful smell and the youngest leaves can be made in to a refreshing summer tea that is delicious hot or cold. It is very calming and will help to ease anxiety and promote restful sleep.

ROSEMARY: will grow to a large shrub if given the room but can be contained to a smaller size if planted in a tub. Bruise a couple of stems and then infuse in sweet almond oil to use either as an invigorating muscle rub or to add to a bath in order to aid relaxation. The evergreen nature of this aromatic shrub means that its health-boosting potential can be accessed at times when other herbs are dormant. As a kitchen herb, its flavour is best incorporated in slow-cooking casseroles, soups and roasts.

THYME: planting a little thyme amongst your vegetables or in a window box will help deter insects and parasites and bring fresh flavour to each meal. Eaten regularly, thyme will give a powerful boost to your own immune system, making it a useful herb during the cold season.

SAGE: this herb has many uses for oral health. It can be steeped in boiled water, left to cool and used as a gargle for soothing a sore throat or as an effective mouthwash. It can be rubbed on to the gums to promote strength or, when eaten, will stimulate digestion, cleanse the blood and balance the hormones.

GERANIUMS: these attractive plants bring joy to any windowsill and their therapeutic effects are an added bonus. Cut up a few leaves and infuse in some oil for a couple of weeks. After this time, you will have an effective remedy for menstrual cramps; simply massage in as needed. Geranium is also known for its ability to balance mind and body; adding a few drops of geranium-infused oil to your bath will help you to unwind and feel revitalized.

Two of the gardener's most notorious adversaries are the slug and his home-owning cousin, the snail. The obvious answer is not to plant their favourite treats in the first place but, if you must have hostas, put them in a tub with a smear of grease around its middle. The slugs and snails won't cross the grease and your plants will be safe. If you need to plant a bed of marigolds to help keep off the whitefly, add a mulch of pine-needles saved from your unsprayed (and so wonderfully-scented) Christmas tree to once again to keep the marauding gastropods at bay. Alternatively, encircling plants with a band of copper placed half a centimetre off the ground level creates a barrier as it carries a minute electrical charge which the slugs won't cross. If none of these methods appeal, good old garlic can be brought into play again as they hate the smell.

Water is the other ingredient essential to life, so ensure a year-round supply to help draw creatures into your garden more readily. Birds especially need water in winter, when their diet is dependent on drier foods (like seeds and nuts) rather than the juicy fruits of summer. A birdbath is the obvious answer, but think about the possibility of a pond, a shallow dish or even just a little hollow, lined with plastic held down by pebbles, to provide a place for refreshment. Even if it takes a season for the locals to discover it, once they have you will be blessed with regular visits from a whole variety of birds and insects. The real joy will come in a couple of seasons' time when your garden is finally clear of any toxic residue and, if you're lucky, along will come a frog or maybe even a hedgehog to keep your slug population under control for you.

Another element to bring to the natural garden is wood. Any old tree that has had to be cut down will soon become host to a whole variety of insects which, if left alone, may eventually include the increasingly rare stag beetle. The beauty and interest of wood and the creatures and fungi that colonize it remind us that even in decay irrepressible nature finds an opportunity for regeneration. Indeed, this is one of the greatest gifts a garden has to offer as it reminds us of the circular nature of life. At times of loss, one can look to nature to remind oneself of rebirth; we see that nothing ends, it merely enters a period of rest before rising up once again, strong and everlasting.

As the growing season draws to a close, remember to leave as many seed-heads on as possible. Their rich nutrients will encourage birds into your garden throughout the winter and then, come spring, the birds will return the favour by picking off the aphids that every garden attracts. For every pest there are at least two or three predators, not just birds but also ladybirds, hover-flies and beetles. From tiny insects to beautiful butterflies and singing birds, the natural garden is alive with activity. The presence of this fervent hum adds a whole new dimension that is entirely lacking from the sterile arena that results from chemical use. Add to that the possibility of other visitors whom you may never actually get to see and the garden starts to resonate with mystery and enchantment.

If you are lucky enough to have larger animals such as deer, foxes or badgers come into your garden, one of the best things you can do for them (particularly in urban areas) is to reinforce the idea that they should avoid humans at all costs. Do not feed them inappropriate food such as that intended for humans or dogs (if it is not organic it will be full of synthetic chemicals) and, if you are lucky enough to make eye-contact with these delightful creatures, savour the blessing and then clap your hands loudly. The next person they meet might not be as nice as you are.

There is nothing to beat the alchemy that takes place in a truly natural garden. No amount of designer decking or planting of exotic sensitives will stimulate the senses like a robust and deliciously fecund, natural garden. If at this time you do not have access to your own, private wonderland, do what you can to foster your connection with nature. Window boxes full of native flowers will still attract butterflies, while feeders hung from brackets will attract birds as surely as the ones hung from trees. An indoor potted fern placed by an open window will rustle as delightfully as any would outside and the growing and eating of just a single pot of herbs is guaranteed to boost both your health and your spirits.

CHAPTER 25

The Turning of the Year

Before the days of central heating and refrigeration, our lives were shaped by the changing seasons. Our dependence on the seasonal ebb and flow was the framework within which the year was played out: the onset of winter, the long slog of survival before the first warm days of spring, the blossoming of summer and the all-important harvest. Just as this seasonal shifting tradition- ally gave form to our lives, so it still gives form to our energies. For we too ebb and flow: with the weather, with the passage of the Sun, with the phases of the Moon and with internal tides so subtle that we barely acknowledge them. If we can re-attune to this waxing and waning, we are apt to find that life flows more easily, with less effort and greater reward.

The cyclical nature of the natural year is the reason for its sustainability; activity without rest leads to exhaustion, just as surely as rest without activity leads to stagnation. In harmony with nature, we humans also follow cycles of action and rest, subconsciously peaking and troughing in a continuous pattern of bio-rhythmical fluctuation. We respond to these cycles through the actions of our hormones, which then initiate various physiological and psy- chological responses. Sometimes external forces instigate these internal reac- tions for example, the lengthening or shortening of the day, which prompts the desire to procreate, hibernate or migrate. Other cycles, such as the 24- hour circadian rhythm, continue regardless of external disruption, which is why jetlag and sleep-deprivation cause such mental and physical distress. Come winter, the seasonal decrease in sunlight finds many people suffering from an increased need for sleep as well as a craving for carbohydrates and a tendency towards social withdrawal. Extreme suffering of these symptoms renders even routine chores difficult to carry out and has now been medically recognized as Seasonal Affective Disorder (SAD Syndrome). However, what is less well-acknowledged is that we are all subject to the instinct to internal- ize our energies in winter, just as the animals hibernate and the trees shed their leaves before blossoming again in spring.

Unfortunately, our 24/7 way of life is leaving us increasingly alienated from our cyclical natures, with both individuals and society beginning to suf- fer under the expectation of 100% energy at all times. A 2002 study (*Britain's World of Work - The Myths and Realities*) by the Economic and Social Research Council[17] has shown that, when employees are continually kept under high pressure to meet targets and appraisals, the outcome is a lowering of morale accompanied by a withdrawal of commitment to the employer. When looked at in terms of energy, this can be viewed as an emotional shutting-down in response to expectations that are energetically unsustainable. Viewed alongside the fact that continued high pressure is known to cause problems for our physical health, it must now be acknowledged that adequate and regular periods of respite are intrinsic to the maintenance of health because they bring balance to the energetic equation. Only by ensuring that time for rest and relaxation is woven in to the fabric of society (in the family, in education and in business) can our personal highs and lows hope to be accommodated. Furthermore, recognizing how subject we are to this energetic ebb and flow allows us to interpret our own and others' behaviour much more effectively, thereby understanding the mood-swings which manifest both within ourselves and within society.

Energy is never static: it is always either expanding outward or contracting inwards, forever in a state of flux. The long days and high temperatures of summer encourage an expansion of energy, both individually and within society. We tend to become more active, to spend more time outdoors and to feel more inclined to socialize. Contrarily, the onset of winter finds us retreating into our homes and ourselves: a physical and mental battening-down of the hatches until spring warms and stirs our spirits. When a hard winter is followed by a late spring, humankind begins to pay dearly for want of active energy. There is a tendency towards depression and lethargy, illness and even death. Life is lived in the moment but continuing life is dependent on the continuation of the energetic cycle, whether that means winter's dormancy, the arrival of spring or the release of the rainy season.

The yin and yang symbol of Feng Shui illustrates this very neatly. The unified whole is only achieved by the presence of two opposing energies: the contracting, cooling, pacifying nature of yin counterbalancing the expanding, heated, active nature of yang. When energy continues either to expand or contract for a sustained period without a counterbalance, there is an inevitable backlash, an implosion or explosion that catapults energy into the opposite state. For example, when a group of individuals gather together, the energy of the self can become sublimated to the external energy of the pack. As this externalized pack-energy amasses, the expanding physical and mental force builds in the form of heat and tension until it eventually over-spills and finds its channel through outgoing, sometimes even aggressive, action. The shock of this outburst fills the individual with fear, the instinct then being to scuttle back behind physical or emotional barriers for a period of introspection until wounds heal and a sense of balance is restored.

On other occasions, energy is externalized as a means of balancing intensely-felt, personal emotions. Attaching rituals to such key moments as the arrival of a new baby, a marriage or the funeral of a loved-one provides us with a framework through which to process our emotional need to believe in something more powerful than ourselves, i.e. to feel cared for and blessed by a benevolent Spirit or God. By expressing such energy out beyond the personal realm and into the collective ether, we give form and flow to our hopes, our fears or our sadnesses. At times of social upheaval, such as war or economic depression, rates of suicide and personal depression tend to decrease. At times like these, people feel connected to one another and can externalize their energy in the collective fight for survival or justice. This counterbalances the raw, personal grief which they may be experiencing and so allows the individual to endure emotional and physical hardships that would seem inconceivable in better times. Over-internalizing sadness means that this energy has nowhere to go, with even some doctors now recognizing that unresolved emotional trauma could be the trigger for killers such as heart disease and cancer.

Getting the balance right is the key to good health and it is here that nature provides the perfect role model; by fully honouring the ebb and flow of the natural year, we reconnect to the energy of the wider rolling world. This in turn helps to draw us out of the introspection that can make a personal crisis seem insurmountable or the ordinary simply mundane. In times of uncertainty or dismay, we are reminded that we are part of a continuum: the Sun will rise again and so will we.

By celebrating the events, seasons and festivals that mark our time on Earth, we not only honour our own gift of life but also our place in the ongoing story of our planet and our cosmos. The energetic release of the festival brings nourishment and joy back into lives that are dominated by routine, encouraging us to come together and recognize life for what it should be: a party. In Europe, the tradition of festivals dates back from before the arrival of the Ancient Romans, with their pantheon of gods and goddesses, to the era of the Celts. Their world was one of trees and weather and seasons and they honoured their interdependence with nature through ritualistic feasts and ceremonies. The language and symbolism of these ancient people was inextricably entwined with the forces of nature and it is a testimony to the depth of their understanding that many of the festivals still being celebrated in homes today have their roots firmly planted in Celtic tradition.

The Celts understood that humankind was but one small part of nature's grand design and that only through careful study, undertaken with deep reverence towards the living Spirit, would they be able to decipher its eternal wisdom. The knowledge which this study garnered was passed down from generation to generation and held in the special care of the wise elders. The Druids were the philosophers of this venerated class; they would advise the tribal leaders in matters of law and judgement. The Ovates were the teachers, responsible for the education of novices at the Druid colleges. Finally, there were the Bards, who would roam the countryside telling stories of their clan's great conquests and wisdom. The power wielded by these philosophers, professors and poets was substantial, sometimes greater than that of the kings themselves but there was always humility before the omnipotent Spirit of Nature. The Celts recognized the ultimate supremacy of Nature and it was this that led them to the practise of deification and worship that survives to this day.

The Celtic year was split into two halves: the dark and the light. Marriage was forbidden during the dark months and, for this reason, many marriages (in the loosest sense) took place with the dawning of the light part of the year: Beltane, or May Day as it's known today. This ancient festival of fertility saw houses being decorated with freshly-cut green branches and flowers to encourage the fertilizing energy of spring into every home in the village. On May Day eve, young couples would pair off, returning at dawn to erect a May pole or felled tree-trunk. This none too subtle representation of the phallic male pole entering yielding Mother Earth was accompanied by symbolic spiral and maypole dancing. A May King and Queen would be crowned and the unbridled merry-making would last for many hours. The energy and passion aroused through such carousing would hope to ensure a bountiful harvest at summer's end.

We too experience a surge of primal energy as May Day welcomes the summer in. With the warmth and heat of the waxing Sun overcoming winter's chill, renewed energy pulses through our veins and sinews. It is a time of great expectancy and vigour, with the whole world seeming to burst with pure potentiality. As the heady scent of spring flowers fills us with its potency, we leave behind the conservatism of winter and become a little wilder in our perceptions of what's possible. Throw open your home, your psyche and your body to all that May brings; the very word expresses possibility, so do all you can to embrace it.

This season's boost of energy makes it the perfect time of year for the traditional spring clean: the grand clear out of all that is of no further use and a thorough overhaul of the rest. Any particularly demanding projects, such as decoration or refurbishment, will be far easier to complete now than in the winter months. Physiological and emotional cobwebs can also be cleared as this is a great time to undertake a detoxification programme, re-start regular exercise and begin munching on all those potent summer salad vegetables. Harness the optimism of this time of year and direct it into the launch of any new ventures or ideas that have been formulating over the winter months. Your energy and expectation of success form the fertile ground upon which new projects or relationships will flourish. Re-establish contacts with friends who may possibly have been hibernating just like you. Throw a party to get the summer going; you never know, you may inspire your friends to do likewise and so make for a sociable summer full of fun and happy memories. Barbecues, picnics and camping all carry with them echoes of times past when our lives were lived much closer to nature. Even the most reluctant of gardeners ventures out to be charmed by nature's magic and en masse we begin to spend more and more time out of doors, availing ourselves of the healing power of the Sun. As the cycle of energetic buoyancy builds, we begin to look and feel better, revitalized from within by the unseen forces of the Universe.

As summer proceeds, this exuberant energy is directed out towards our friends, family and all manner of personal and professional projects and, by the season's climax, we begin to see the fruits of our labours. In the days of the Celts, this time of harvest was celebrated with the festival of Lughnassadh, which symbolized the marrying of the god Lugh to the Mother Earth. By bestowing honour on Mother Earth, these celebrations hoped to ensure her continued benevolence come the following spring. Lammas is another incarnation of this festival, dating from medieval times and celebrated on the same day, August 1st. The word Lammas is derived from the Anglo-Saxon word 'hlafmaesse' meaning loaf mass; it relates to the breaking of freshly-baked bread made from the newly-harvested grain. Other festivities included the making of corn dolls, the drinking of whisky made from barley and of beer made from hops. Deliciously nutritious fruits and berries were also gathered at this time and are still to be found in abundance in the late summer hedgerows of today. Their rich vitamin and mineral content continues to boost immune systems preparing to face the rigours of winter, with any surplus being preserved in jams and pickles ready for the months ahead. Celebrate this time of harvest by planning a late summer picnic incorporating all the fruits of this time of year, at least some of which can hopefully come from your own garden: pickles with cheese, bread and preserves, muffins and summer puddings, all washed down with beer or cider. Make the most of the now-waning Sun by continuing to spend time outdoors. Notice which flowers are coming into late bloom and which are morphing into hips and berries. Often, it is only as things begin to fade that they are truly appreciated, so learn this lesson with each passing season and soon you will begin to relish every moment, trusting the future to look after itself.

The finale of the growing season is a flamboyant splash of autumnal colour: the reds, golds and oranges that signal the shedding of this year's growth in preparation for the coming spring's renewal. As the falling leaves return to their roots, their decay forms a protective bed of rich humus, which in turn provides a supply of nutrition to the parent plant and shelter to animals preparing to hibernate. The Celts intuitively understood this cycle of decay and renewal and celebrated it with the autumn festival of Samhain. Beginning at sundown on October 31st, the festivities bore witness to the death of the Old Year and continued until sunrise the following day, whereupon the New Year would be welcomed in. As the winter Moon sought ascendancy over the waning summer Sun, Samhain represented a time of reckoning, when ancestral spirits were invoked to bring guidance and resolution to any disputes within the clan. Being once again at peace with one another meant that the community was better able to survive the journey into the dark months ahead. Fires would be lit against the encroaching darkness and the clan would gather together to ask for the protection of their ancestors and safe deliverance into the waiting arms of spring. When the Christians arrived, they recognized that so strong was this tradition, their only hope was to commandeer it by making it hallowed or holy, and claiming it as the day for all their saints.

We too bring fire into our lives at this time of year, especially in Britain where, every November 5th, millions of us gather around communal bonfires to pierce the autumnal darkness with light. Although this festival supposedly remembers the deeds of one Guy Fawkes, it seems strange that a relatively obscure historic event should provoke such a powerful and ongoing communal response. It is far more likely that we are responding to the primal memory of the fire festival of Samhain. To this day, we submit to the urge to leave our homes and make our last stance against the onset of winter. Warmed by spiced wines or hot buttered rum and heartened by traditional foods such as baked potatoes, sausages and soup, family, friends and neighbours huddle together under starry skies to gaze transfixed at the magnificence of the bonfire. With such elemental forces around, it's no wonder that thoughts become reflective and hearts sincere.

As the nights draw in, we close our curtains on the darkening world and seek to make ourselves cosy and warm by the light of the family fire. In perfect harmony with Nature, we humans experience a turning inward of energy at this time, feeling less inclined to go out socializing and preferring instead to bed-down earlier and sleep longer. With coats wrapped around us and heads bowed against the rain, we battle against the winter weather just as we've always done. It's a very long road ahead til spring; what we need is a party!

Imagine winter without Christmas. Forget the avarice, the gluttony, the pressure to spend, spend, spend. These are all recent manifestations borne out of our society's having too much money and too little imagination. Just imagine, though, winter without Christmas .

The original midwinter festival has nothing to do with the birth of Christ. This was simply another ruse of the early Christians to commandeer Celtic fun in the hope of garnering a few converts. In fact, this ritualistic brightening of the darkest days of the year is as much a part of our pre-Christian heritage as bonfire night. By comparing the simple pleasure associated with that night to the insanity of a modern Christmas, we see how we have been manipulated. For, despite the fact that many of the traditions associated with Christmas date back to the time of the Celts, commercialism and consumerism have conspired to eclipse almost entirely the more natural and spiritual aspects of this festival. Nevertheless, even the most cynical of non-believers still responds to the impulse to shed light into the wintry darkness and, fortunately, there are plenty of ways in which to celebrate without ever resorting to shiny new baubles, soon-to-be-redundant gizmos or frozen, factory-farmed turkey.

The original midwinter festival began on the night of winter's solstice, December 21st, and it celebrated the rebirth of the Sun after its symbolic death during the shortest day of the year. The traditions and rituals performed at this time honoured the continuing cycle of life, death and rebirth, a concept perfectly embodied in the festive wreath which to this day is displayed decorated with leaves, acorns, pine cones, mistletoe and berries, just as it was then. Struggling through the dark months of winter, the return of the warmth and light meant the difference between life and death to the Celts, so a Yule Log would be lit on midwinter's eve and kept burning throughout the festivities, its fire acting as an enticement to the reluctant Sun. Once burnt out, its ashes would then be scattered across the fields in the hope of procuring a fertile spring. In the modern home, not only will a chocolate-covered Yule Log cake make a more traditional centre-piece than marzipan and fruitcake, but wood can be burnt in the fireplace (if permitted), its ash then 'offered' to the compost heap ready to enrich the Earth with potash come springtime. Today, the Sun's warmth can be further wooed by lighting candles and using dried slices of orange and bunches of red, yellow or orange chillies as decoration.

Evergreens were traditionally cut and hung about the house to represent the enduring spirit of nature: holly for endurance and ivy conveying resilience in the face of winter. If mistletoe, then known as All Heal, was found growing in the boughs of an oak tree, the Celts considered it very auspicious indeed as it was believed to contain the fertile life-essence of its majestic host. Today, mistletoe reveals itself as one of the most powerful healers in the natural apothecary, increasingly recognized for its ability to fight cancer. If possible, grow these plants in your own garden for their year-round beauty and their ability to brighten the home come midwinter. Pot up early-flowering bulbs such as cyclamen, snowdrops and even hyacinths to bring further decoration into your home. Once the festivities are over, they can then be planted out in the garden or stored ready for next year. Many people are now turning away from using a natural tree. However, as long as you ensure that your real, unsprayed tree is recycled, it is still an eco-friendly option when compared to the environmental costs of manufacturing a synthetic one. To decorate your tree, suspend gerberas or chrysanthemums in their own little test-tubes of water, tie bundles of cinnamon sticks with ribbons, hang clusters of berries and citrus slices pierced with cloves to all bring colour to the branches without resorting to environmentally-damaging baubles. As a final touch, sprays of gypsophila lain over the branches of the tree will give a much more naturalistic impression of frost than tinsel ever will.

The bounties of Mother Earth were also remembered in festival foods, bought out to honour our hostess and encourage further harvests. Apples, berries, nuts and treats were offered in the hope that giving would encourage receiving. The exchange of presents has got a little out of hand these days, but when gifts have true use and meaning and are not excessive to the receiver's needs or the giver's bank balance, the ritual retains its healthy roots and confers honour on both. The other great tradition associated with this festival is the playing of parlour games. Originally, the Celts devised these games as a means of divining the future. A nut would be tossed onto the fire in response to a specific question; if it popped, the answer was yes, while the lack of a pop meant no. To this day, the yearly appearance of the board-game and annual attempt at charades is an important element in many family Christmases which, together with singing, dancing and general merry-making, all serves to drive away the winter blues, bringing light and joy to the darkest of seasons.

Once the festivities of midwinter are over, we look up and, lo and behold! the days are perceptibly longer. The weather may be as harsh, but the first brave flowers are already raising their heads to encourage us on through the last cold days til spring. However, we are not out of the woods just yet; as the last weeks of winter mingle with the first weeks of spring, a mighty tug-of-war of weather takes place. There can be warmth and sunshine in February and biting winds and driving snow in March. For the Celts, as for animals and for modern people, these last, almost excruciating days of winter can mean the difference between continuing life and the death of this life. In the time of the Celts, an effigy of the green man would be sacrificed, symbolizing the shedding of the old, worn-out physical skin to make way for spiritual re-birth. Today, the annual rise in mortality rates seen at this time of year is rationalized as the result of cold weather and lowered immunity but, in these days of flu jabs, central heating and year-round availability of food, is it not perhaps possible that we are answering to a more ancient call?

Whatever the weather is doing, the days are growing longer and the Sun rides higher in the sky. The Celtic festival of this time was known as Imbolc (from 'oimelc', meaning 'sheep's milk') and symbolizes the new-born taking nourishment from the mother figure. This festival welcomed the now strongly-waxing Sun and glorified the Triple goddess Brigid, who gave the festival its other name of Brigantia. The multiple form of this goddess as virgin, matron and crone evokes the season's progress at a time when the seemingly-lifeless gives birth to new growth. As spring energizes the reflective thoughts of winter, true wisdom manifests and, for the Celts, the resulting ability to shed light on the unseen was represented by the willow tree and the Moon, which together ruled the month of February. These very feminine influences found their expression through seership, which is the divination of truth through dreams and night visions. Whilst the monthly cycle of the

Moon has long been known to reflect the female cycle of fertility, the ability of the willow to drive the agues and suffering out of a person has found modern affirmation now that it is used in medicinal preparations against the damp and discomfort that can cause us such pain.

Perhaps unsurprisingly, the timing of this festival coincides with the Christian festival of Candlemas which occurs on February 2nd and which honours their own female goddess, mother and maiden: the Virgin Mary. However, many of the rituals of this time are more apparent today in the lunar-determined festival of Easter, a name which is itself derived from that of the Anglo-Saxon goddess, Oestra, said to govern this time of year. The most obvious symbol associated with this goddess and her festival is the egg, which neatly sums up the conundrum of re-birth by posing the question: which came first, the chicken or the egg? The Easter bunnies of our greetings cards may have originally been hares, pagan messengers capable of travelling between this world and that of the spirit, drawing down messages from the Moon goddess to the Earth. And whilst the cross has an obviously strong connection to Christianity's own take on life after death, its existence pre-dates Christianity, possibly emulating the ancient Egyptian symbol of life: the Ankh. In the Celtic tradition, the cross couples the female circle with the male cross; a union which is also represented in the circular hot cross buns of our present-day Easter celebrations.

By the time of the spring equinox in March, the feminine power of the Moon has come into perfect harmony with that of the male Sun and it was this marriage of male and female that provided the perfect recipe for healthy reproduction: the harbinger of a fruitful spring.

The potent symbiosis of intuitive, creative, female energy with the fiery, ardent male is a marriage of cosmic implications. Honour this time by welcoming the magic of life into your heart and home. Breathe in all that this life-force bestows and simply allow yourself to be awed and amazed by the miracle of nature. Artificial symbols are not needed, for all about us is affirmation of our faith in the benevolent Spirit of Creation. Our trust is rewarded everywhere we look, as out from the dark Earth come the green shoots of life reborn.

CHAPTER 26

The Cosmos

The number three has long been associated with earthly and spiritual incarnations of power hence there were great triumvirates of Ancient Roman rule; the Christian worship of the Father, the Son and the Holy Spirit; and the three chief Gods of Hinduism: Brahma, Vishnu and Shiva. Our own, present-day political system is a triumvirate comprising the Sovereign, the House of Lords and the House of Commons but how did this notion of the ruling three originate? It may well have something to do with the relationship between our own planet and her two nearest neighbours, the Sun and the Moon, for here we see the original and grandest triumvirate of them all. The Sun, giver of light and warmth without which there would be no life; the fertile Earth, which incubates and gives birth to a myriad of life-forms and the mysterious Moon, whose subtle influence governs the unseen cycles and rhythms of our world.

Ever since humankind began to consciously court nature, it has been in the thrall of these stupendous forces and their ability to affect all aspects of our lives: the length of the day, the duration of the growing season, the fruition of the harvest and the turning of the tides. Such was the extent of this influence that, for the last four-and-a-half thousand years, humankind has been observing and analysing the positions, movements and apparent coincidences that give form to our Universe. In 2000 BC Babylon, fascination with the skies led to the first observations ever recorded, thus beginning the scientific study which eventually led to the development of astronomy. The ancient, megalithic monument at Stonehenge dates from a similar period and has been found to have numerous alignments with the Sun and Moon, allowing celestial events to be predicted with an accuracy not equalled until 1000 years later in classical Greece. By the early centuries AD, complicated systems based on mathematical knowledge and empirical evidence increased humankind's understanding and fascination in equal measure. Grecian scholars studied the Earth's shadow on the Moon and were led to surmise the spherical nature of our planet. Timing the duration of eclipses allowed them to calculate that the Earth was approximately three times bigger than the Moon (the actual figure is 3.66 times). In Central America, the Mayan astronomers of 1000 years ago built up such precise observations of eclipses that they were able to predict their recurrence with amazing accuracy. The many Sun- and Moon-dedicated temples, pyramids and observational structures that survive to the present day are testimony to the incredible impact that these heavenly bodies had on the lives of earlier mortals; even today, despite all of our apparent sophistication, the very human response to the Heavens remains one of awe.

For those lucky enough to have looked through a telescope, the sudden realization that, for all its immense beauty, deep space is a cold, dark and seemingly life-lorn place can come as an emotional jolt. It brings into sharp focus the uniqueness of our own planet and its ability to support a range of life-forms as diverse as the great whales of the oceans and the giraffes of the African plains. Here on Earth, the notion of being alone is quite literally alien, surrounded as we are by teeming life that bursts forth at every opportunity. This immense, benevolent Being absorbs our whims and provides us with all we need, her beauty only accentuated by the spectacular passage of the Sun and the gentle gaze of the Moon.

As we humans seek to star in our own tragi-comedy, their steady presence takes us beyond our personal drama to the eternal theatre of the Universe. Within your own personal piece of space, take time out from the manmade histrionics of relationships, religion, politics and responsibilities and simply feel their energy: beneath your feet, on your skin and in your heart. Take the soil in your hands, walk barefoot on the grass, feel the rocks beneath your feet so that you make contact with the true nature of our beautiful planet. Know when the Moon is full, new, waxing or waning and use the energetic influence she brings to plan, consolidate or harvest personal and professional projects. Note the path of the Sun and orientate your rooms so that activity areas are bathed in as much light as possible. Breakfast with the rising Sun, create and realize in the clarity of midday's brightness, meditate and ruminate in the twilight of another day's passing. Bathe in their light; let the Sun warm your body and the Moon illuminate your soul. Be emotionally, even physically naked before the heavens and experience the exhilaration and healing that this brings.

Use colours inspired by the planets to bring natural harmony into the home. The earthiness of ochre, umber and sienna bring grounding to rooms and furnishings, whilst the gold, orange, crimson and violet that suffuse a sunrise bring vibrancy and highlight. The opalescent shimmer of the Moon finds expression through the use of mirrors, glazes, crystal and water; their ability to reflect and refract remind us that what can be seen may not always be touched and that what is felt is not always seen.

Finally always remember the relevance of the number three. For it is only with the addition of the third point that a line becomes a shape and it is only by journeying into the third dimension that shape takes on a solid form. What this tells us is that, whilst the two most powerful players in our triumvirate may appear to be the Sun and the Earth, it is perhaps the presence of the third entity, the Moon, that provides the key to our understanding.

By metaphorically taking us into the third dimension, the presence of the

Moon acknowledges our intuitive feeling that there is an as yet undefined aspect to the human experience. For centuries, humankind has recognized the fact that something else is going on apart from that which can be physically verified. We feel and experience things which cannot be seen or explained and talk about our intuitions as a; 'feeling in our water' the element ruled by the Moon. Unfortunately, this universal insight has long been ignored by the Earth-bound thinking of those who dominate the science of our time. As they seek to expose, dissect and compartmentalize life on Earth, scientists have left the unseen to the seekers of spiritual truths, thus fostering the splitting of the physical and the spiritual which has blinded us to the true explanation for our failing health and emotional unhappiness.

Just because the scientists have analysed and labelled everything to the nth degree does not mean that they have grasped the whole truth. Truth, as it is presented to us, is a shifting dynamic and no one displays this anomaly better than the scientists themselves. Whatever field they are practising in, it seems that they (of all people) are the most likely to get stuck in a particular perspective and thenceforth only be able to interpret what they see in accordance with it. This frequently-observed phenomenon was first highlighted by the U.S. historian and philosopher, Thomas Kuhn. In his 1962 work, *The Structure of Scientific Revolutions*, he argued that prevailing social and cultural conditions direct the course of scientific research. The resulting paradigm then informs scientific knowledge by becoming the dominant theoretical framework. In fact, this knowledge simply represents a series of conjectures and refutations designed to confirm or refute the prevailing ethos. One should therefore always be wary of any dogma (be it scientific, political or religious) for, in effect, it hinders the understanding and wisdom which come from true insight.

While conventional science slowly plods up numerous blind alleys, blinkered by personal arrogance and commercial greed, society persists in seeing itself in accordance with pre-existing doctrines, self-imposed boundaries and generally low expectations. Until we can free ourselves of the strait-jacket of these predetermined projections, we will continue to believe what we are told and deny what we know. Fortunately, just occasionally, insight bursts through and in doing so allows humankind to take a leap forward. Freedom, if only we know how to ask for it, can then be ours for the taking .

❀ ❀ ❀ The Self / The Whole ❀ ❀ ❀

To this day, our society's framework remains largely based on the ideas put forward by the 17th century English physicist and mathematician, Isaac Newton. In discovering that white light was composed of many colours and in developing both the law of gravity and the three laws of motion still in use today, his work laid the foundations of physics as a modern, scientific discipline. His contribution was so immense that society became (and has remained) entrenched in his point of view, one which saw our world as being made up of solid building blocks of matter. As his theories were developed by further generations of Newtonian physicists, the physical world was broken down into atoms, the smallest unit capable of taking part in a chemical reaction. Each atom was found to contain indivisible positive and negative electrical charges (known as protons and electrons respectively) as well as neutrons, which contain a similar mass to protons but have no charge. These particles were interpreted as being essentially solid and mechanical in nature, thereby allowing everything to be explained in strictly causal terms. Space and time were absolute and linear. All was objectively measurable.

This neat rationale persists in the language which we use to describe our world and ourselves to this day. Despite living in a sceptical age, our tendency is still to trust what we are told over what we may feel or intuit. Our actual experience is harnessed and interpreted by the mechanics of the ticking clock and by a system of expectations that is ingrained in us from childhood. Seeking meaning from within this mechanistic framework allows us to reclaim that which is not easily understood and reassures us about probable outcomes and reactions. Unfortunately, it is our dependence on this framework that prevents us from embracing more intuitive insights and deciphering their messages.

Whilst individuals and society continue in the main to accept this mechanical interpretation of events, physics as a science has moved on. The discovery of electromagnetism in the early 19th century propelled thinking in the direction of a totally new concept, that of the field. Rather than the fixed notions of the Newtonians, this new thinking focused less on matter and more on energetic charge, force and disturbance. It inferred that the Universe, and all within it, are comprised of interacting fields of force which are electrical, magnetic or gravitational in nature. As people are part of this Universal field, they both influence and are influenced by its forces, which are experienced as being either harmonious or disruptive. This new insight made sense of many previously inexplicable human experiences whereby intuitions about people, situations and places had caused a feeling later borne out by experience.

It also implied that the energy of an individual could, and always would, influence the outcome of any given event.

To add to this burgeoning worldview came Albert Einstein. In 1905, his Special Theory of Relativity unleashed a concept that, at least as far as theoretical physics was concerned, blew away the last vestiges of Newtonian thinking. Einstein theorized that space and time were not in fact absolute and linear but relative to one another and taken together form the fourth dimension necessary to our understanding of space and time. The idea that time and space are not, in fact, absolute perplexes logical, mechanical thinking but causes our intuitive selves to leap for joy. It explains the numerous incidences of premonitions, visions, déjà vu and other lapses in the apparent time continuum when the world is glimpsed out of synch. Even on the most mundane level, many people will recognize time's capacity to fly when they are having fun but to drag its feet interminably when they are bored. The very well-known expression 'a watched kettle never boils' puts these experiences at the heart of our culture, yet society still seeks to rationalize its existence within the confines of Newtonian cause and effect rather than interpreting life according to reality as it is experienced.

Every time science believes that it has it all wrapped up, some tiny part of the equation slips through the scientist's fingers and nature retains its mystery. By the 1920s, the paradoxical nature of the sub-atomic world, where light had been proven to be both particle and wave in form, caused scientists to identify energy packets, which they termed 'quanta'. These quanta replaced the previous definition of particles, allowing quantum theory to sweep away all previous notions of matter, mass and elementary particles under the new realization that all was, in fact, energy and as such infinitely transmutable. The possibility that matter could both manifest and vanish back into the energetic field confounds the lay person's understanding of the physical world. For we now see that nothing is solid, fixed or predetermined as was first believed; instead, there are infinite possible outcomes, with at most a tendency towards a particular event's happening, which may then manifest a particular effect or not.

If this is the nature of the sub-atomic world then it is surely the nature of our world, too. By beginning to think in terms of tendencies rather than in terms of facts, the sheer possibility of all that is available to us becomes clear. In any given scenario, there are an infinite number of possible outcomes and potential realities for us to choose from. Where there is the possibility of anger, there is the possibility of understanding. Which do we choose to manifest? Where there is the potential for health, there is also the potential for dis-ease; which do we allow to dominate our lives? Do we radiate harmony or dis-harmony from our personal field into the universal field? Choices like these, often made in the smaller moments of our lives, ultimately create our own, uniquely personal life-experience. Our view of the world and subsequent interpretations of it become shaped by our dominant mode of reaction: namely, love or fear. Only by reassessing our mode of reaction can conscious thought be brought into the frame, thereby allowing us to re-evaluate the nature of our reality.

In accepting that we are ultimately responsible for our own reality, we must also accept that we have no one to blame or thank but ourselves. The usual, immediate and Newtonian response to this is that it is our birthplace and situation that have the primary influence on all subsequent opportunities and experiences. But at what point does the choosing and manifesting begin? If life is not simply about physical matter but something more intangible and elusive, then does this not imply that creation is about more than just the meeting of sperm and ova? The primal urge to procreate and the all-powerful need to ensure the survival of the species comes from where, exactly?

Whilst the spiritual thinkers and theoretical scientists ponder the question of where we come from, we, as individuals, tend to focus on the here and now, vaguely aware that there is perhaps one factor above others that influences our experience: our health. In their early years, most people take this for granted; a predisposition towards good health is, after all, the pre-requisite of a successful species. However, as one gets older, things become a little more complex and, in time, our faith in our physical selves comes to be tested. At such times, we can gain strength from the knowledge that holistic health, of which physical wellbeing is but one part, flows from a source far deeper than that addressed by the present, mechanistic model of healthcare. No one set of circumstances ever truly mimics another, so the use of fixed treatments and prognoses loses it validity. Rather, healthcare is about the interaction and interpretation of many factors and the possibility of many outcomes. This state of being is not fixed and nothing, not history and certainly not the future, is carved in stone or summed up in probability-factors. What we have to remember above all else is that we have influence at a very personal and individual level. Healing journals are full of examples of people who have confounded doctors' expectations by using techniques such as transcendental meditation, exercise, changes in lifestyle, nutrition, visualization, affirmations and other methods of investment in the self in order to access their own innate ability to heal. This indicates that something beyond pills and potions is at work. By choosing wholeheartedly to take control of the healing process, either by going outside the prevailing doctrine or by supporting conventional treatment with their own, conscious mental and physical input it appears that a person creates the intention to become well and wellness follows.

It is by focusing our attention on our *intention* that we find the key to accessing our true power, because our intention is the trigger that creates all future manifestations. When wishing to turn to the right, a person simply has to have that intention and their physical bodies do what's necessary to complete the turn. When wishing to impress, the intention to do so creates changes in facial expression, voice pattern, body language and energy field. If somebody takes a placebo pill believing that it is intended to cure their ulcer, their body will initiate the healing of that ulcer. We do not need to mechanically instigate such behaviour because the intention to do so is enough to cause these radically differing physiological, emotional and energetic changes.

Having recognized the power of intention in any given scenario, issues that have been holding us back for years can begin to be resolved. Do we allow ourselves to continue as we have been or do we intend to change? Do we remain sad, angry or defensive or do we envisage another future for ourselves and take steps towards our intended place of arrival? Our future health and happiness is our own responsibility but if we absolve ourselves of our accountability, we give the reins of our lives to others, thereby undermining the essence of the human experience: that of self-determination. If, instead, we choose to act 'in good faith', out of a sense of what is right in Spirit rather than simply taking the route of least responsibility or care, then we can begin to initiate healing at the most fundamental level of our existence.

Despite the millions of man-hours and billions of dollars spent on theoretical and practical research, it seems that our present economic, political and social policy is causing humankind to travel towards energetic chaos rather than harmony. Our race to find answers to the true nature of creation has been paralleled by an era of unprecedented destruction. As our development and use of technology becomes more sophisticated, it is being used to hasten the devastation of our planet through intensive exploitation of natural resources, ecosystems, animals, even humankind itself. Despite this rampaging abuse of the natural world, half of the world's population is dying for want of the basic necessities while the other half faces an epidemic of obesity and addiction. The more we have, the greater our fear of loss; the ensuing combination of fear and pride leads rulers to invest in the instruments of protectionism and war. Now, as the most powerful nation on Earth spends billions in waging a war of ideology, a chasm is appearing in the very fabric of our existence. With the world plummeting into deepening crisis, it is the dark side of possibility that is being manifested rather than the light. It is for us as individuals to ask why and what we can do about it.

In the face of such entrenched destructiveness, the actions of an individual seem unlikely to instigate global reform, but the fact is that there is no such thing as an individual, for we are all constituent parts of a much greater whole. Just as the individual cells of the body join others to form tissues, which then join others still to form bones, which then join yet more to form the skeleton, so an individual joins others to form a family which then joins others to form a community, which then joins others to form a society. And, just as in any family, what affects one affects all.

In 1964, the physicist J.S. Bell mathematically proved a connection between all sub-atomic particles. This connection appears to transcend space and time, allowing effects to be transmitted at superluminal speeds, i.e. faster than the speed of light. This mathematical theory has been observed in countless empirical studies and explains how certain ideas or concepts (such as fashion crazes, crowd behaviour or ideologies) seem to appear from nowhere to spread like wildfire. One such observation was made shortly after the Second World War and it came to the attention of a wider audience through the writings of Lyall Watson in his book, *Lifetide: a Biology of the Unconscious* (Sceptre,1987). In this book, he refers to a scientific study of a group of island-dwelling monkeys in Japan. To attract them on to the beach for the purposes of observation, the scientists left sweet potatoes for the monkeys to eat. However, sand would soon cover the potatoes and the monkeys would not then eat them. Eventually, a resourceful young monkey had the intelligence to wash the potatoes in a stream, rendering them edible. Soon, all the younger monkeys were following suit. This same enterprizing spirit then realized that saltwater further improved the flavour of the vegetable and, before long, a significant proportion of the group was washing its food in the sea. One evening, the number of monkeys displaying this behaviour seemed to have crossed some kind of significant threshold and suddenly all the remaining monkeys simultaneously adopted the practice. This would be interesting in itself but what was truly remarkable was that this newly-adopted behaviour seemingly jumped across natural barriers and spontaneously showed up in other colonies at great distances from the original troop. Watson termed the apparently miraculous ability of behavioural trends to transcend time and distance 'The Hundredth Monkey Phenomenon'. This phenomenon has been seen many times and not just in animal behaviour. Similar breakthroughs in technology frequently emerge from different corners of the world at the same time. The race to patent new ideas and the secrecy in which research is carried out is a testament to this phenomenon. The question is whether this represents truly new behaviour or whether these individual actions key in to an already existing field of intelligence that carries with it all we need to know for our survival. Could it be that, once this intelligence has been accessed or initiated by the actions of enough individuals, it then becomes readily available to the masses?

In his book, *A New Science of Life: The Hypothesis of Morphic Resonance* (Inner Traditions International, 1995), the biologist Rupert Sheldrake proposes the existence of invisible fields of intelligent organization which regulate the physical, behavioural and social actions and interactions of everything from individual atoms to global ecosystems. These morphic fields carry the

the collected, evolutionary memory of every organism and species, allowing for the cohesive organization of each actual, physical unit be that a molecule, an animal or an ecosystem. This, argues Sheldrake, is why, despite all the cells of an organism carrying the same DNA, some cells know to become muscle and some to become bone, why termites know to build nests and birds know to migrate. In terms of societies, the organization of behaviour, theory and language gives coherence to group practice thus allowing religious, political, economic, scientific or social doctrines to come to be perceived as the norm (as recognized by Thomas Kuhn), when in truth what they represent is merely the norm for now. This newly-normalized behaviour then remains entrenched until an apparently spontaneous leap in creative thinking occurs, such as with the genius of the potato-washing monkey. If this new or modified behaviour is accepted and repeated a resonance builds, eventually becoming substantial enough to affect the field of that whole species, thereby creating a new norm. What this tells us is that what may at first appear as individual genius in fact represents the precursor to an intellectual, moral or spiritual leap forward in the collective intelligence of the species. Because this effect occurs at superluminal speed, it appears to transcend the usual linear methods of speech and sight.

The potential for change is therefore always upon us because we can choose whether to reaffirm the present norm or to create a new one. Having recognized that we, too, are part of this all-embracing sea of intelligence that carries with it the ability to organize and harmonize every aspect of life, we can begin to change our world. Just as we continually send and receive information on a cellular level within the physical body, so we continually send and receive intelligence and information between people and organisms outside of our bodies; information that is not constrained by language, geography or even time. In the Universal field of all possibilities, we can choose whether to accept the status quo and allow ourselves to be carried by the tidal influences of others or to throw our own pebbles in and create a new, more harmonious resonance.

The future is ours to shape, but only by taking the reins of responsibility back into our own hands can we hope to influence the world towards a brighter future. Whenever we make a choice whether it's the decision to purchase this product over that, to insist or to acquiesce, to allow our compassion or our ego to drive us we send a resonating vibration out into the energetic field of the entire planet. Any decision, even an apparently insignificant one, sets in motion a wave of resonance that, if it meets another similar resonance, could ultimately culminate in sufficient momentum to turn the tide of communal thinking. This is what we have to remember when we are in the shops and markets choosing non-toxic, fairly-traded and cruelty-free products.

This is why it is imperative that we speak up when those in power act flagrantly against the collective good of humankind. This is why we must put our money where are mouths are and reclaim the future for the good of all. For we do not exist in an individual vacuum, we co-exist in an eternally interacting field of being. We cannot harm others, be they fellow humans, animal life or plant life without hurting ourselves. Inaction is not an option because we are intimately involved at a far deeper level than we seem willing to acknowledge at present. We have the responsibility and the power to bring about change on both a personal and a global level and the place to begin is with the small but multitudinous decisions that give shape to our homes and our lives.

So, next time you are making choices whether it is over which cleaning product or chocolate to buy, or whether to take control of your own life or show concern for another's make kindness your intention. Choose compassionately and every time you do you will reaffirm your connection to humankind, to nature, to the Earth and to the unseen Spirit that unites us. The World Health Organization recognizes that health is more than just the absence of disease or disability, it is about physical, emotional and, crucially, social wellbeing. So, put light behind your thinking in everything you do and say. Be kind to yourself and to others, decide to be healthy and empower your every action with conscious thought. Remember that positive, life-affirming action does just that: it affirms life. Only when we achieve the peace and serenity that come from living honestly, with absolute respect for the inherent connection that exists between ourselves and all other living things, can we attain this state of true, holistic health. It isn't hard and you don't need to wait for everyone else to be doing it before it becomes worthwhile. It just takes enough of us to care sufficiently about our holistic, global home for humankind to finally make the leap forward to a place we've previously only dreamed of .

POSTSCRIPT

Thanks to the efforts of many, new developments are continually being made in the fields of complementary healthcare, ethical trade and environmentally-sustainable technology. I would like to thank all the people and organisations listed on the following pages for their help and continued campaigning for the benefit of us all.

Appendices

REFERENCES

1. US Environmental Protection Agency: Questions About Your Community Indoor Air. Boston, June 2004
2. Dr Michael Cork: The rising prevalence of atopic eczema and environmental trauma to the skin'. *Dermatology in Practice* Vol. 10 No.3, 2002
3. Michael Farthing: COPE Editorial *Gut online* 44:1-1, January 1999
4. Terry Marsden and Nicholas Parrott: *Real Green Revolution*, Greenpeace Environmental Trust, London, February 2002
5. Louise Newman: *British Lifestyles Report*, Mintel, 2005
6. World Trade Co-operative Bank Ethical Policy Unit, Manchester, 2002
7. Oxfam International: *Rigged Rules and Double Standards*, 2002
8. Peter Hardstaff and Tim Jones: *Treacherous Conditions Report*. World Development Movement, London, May 2003
9. J.Madeley: *Crops and Robbers: 5 case studies of poor farmers and communities whose livelihoods are threatened by patenting*. ActionAid, October 2001
10. Oxfam: *Mugged*, 2003
11. UN Food and Agriculture Organization: *Forest Resources Assessment 2000*, Main Report (FRA 2000). FAO Forestry Paper 140, Rome, 2001
12. Working Group 2: *Impacts, Adaptation and Vulnerability*; Intergovernmental Panel on Climate Change, 2001
13. Jonathan Loh and Mathis Wackernagel: *Living Planet Report*, World Wildlife Fund, Switzerland, 2004
14. Philip Lymbery: *Farm Assurance Schemes and Animal Welfare - Can We Trust Them?* Compassion In World Farming, 2002
15. Heather Pickett and Kerry Burgess: Supermarkets and Farm Animal Welfare, *Raising the Standard' Survey 2003-2004*. Compassion in World Farming, 2004
16. Roslyn McKendry: *Home and Garden Survey*, Pesticide Action Network, London, December 2002
17. Robert Taylor: *Britain's World of Work - the Myths and Realities*, Economic and Social Research Council, 2002

BIBLIOGRAPHY

Birren, Faber: *Color Theory And Color Psychology*. Citadel Press, New Jersey. 1979

Emoto, Dr Masaru: *Messages from Water Vol.1*, Beyond Words Publishing, Portland, Oregon. 1999

Humphrys, John: *The Great Food Gamble*, Hodder and Stoughton, London. 2001

Kuhn, Thomas: *The Structure of Scientific Revolutions*, University of Chicago Press. 1962

Ransom, Steve: *Great News on Cancer in the 21st Century*, Credence Publications, Tonbridge. 2002

Sheldrake, Rupert: *A New Science of Life: The Hypothesis of Morphic Resonance*, Inner Traditions International. 1995

Watson, Lyall: *Lifetide: a Biology of the Unconscious*, Sceptre. 1987

USEFUL ADDRESSES

ActionAid International
Post Net Suite248
Private Bag x31, Saxonwold 2132
Johannesburg, South Africa
Tel: +27 11 88 00008
Tel: +27 11 88 08082
www.actionaid.org

ActionAid International UK
Hamlyn House, MacDonald Road
London N19 5PG, UK
Tel: +44 (0) 207 561 7613
www.actionaid.org.uk

Anti-Slavery International
Thomas Clarkson House
The Stableyard, Broomgrove Road
London SW19 9TL, UK
Tel:+44 (0) 20 7501 8920
www.antislavery.org

**BUAV (British Union for the
Abolition of Vivisection)**
16a Crane Grove
London N7 8NN, UK
Tel: + 44 (0) 020 7700 4888
www.buav.org

Campaign for Truth in Medicine
PO Box 3, Tonbridge,
Kent TN12 9zy
Tel: +44 (0) 1622 832 386
www.campaignfortruth.com

**Compassion In World Farming
Compassion In World Farming Trust**
Charles House
5a Charles Street, Petersfield
Hampshire GU32 3EH, UK
Tel: + 44 (0) 1730 268070
www.ciwf.org.uk

The Co-operative Bank
PO Box 101
1Balloon Street
ManchesterM60 4EP, UK
Tel: 08457 212 212
www.cooperativebank.co.uk

Ethical Marketing Group
Publishers of
The GOOD SHOPPING GUIDE
(ISBN 0954 2529 6 9)
105 Westbourne Grove
London W2 4UW
Tel: +44 (0) 207 229 1894
www.ethica-company-organisation.org
www.thegoodshoppingguide.co.uk

Fairtrade Foundation
Suite 204, 16 Baldwin's Gardens
London EC1N 7RJ, UK
www.fairtrade.org.uk

**Fairtrade Labelling Organisations
Worldwide (FLO)**
Kaiser Friedrich Strasse 13
D53113 Bonn, Germany
Tel: +49 228 949 2311
www.fairtrade.net

Oxfam GB
274 Banbury Road
Oxford OX2 7DZ, UK
www.oxfam.org

Pesticide Action Network (PAN) UK
Development House
56-64 Leonard Street
London EC2 4JX, UK
Tel: +44 (0)207 065 0905
www.pan-uk.org
www.pan-international.org
www.pesticidedisposal.org

Pets As Therapy
3 Grange Farm Cottages
Wycombe Road
Saunderton, Princes Risborough
Buckinghamshire HP27 9NS, UK
Tel: +44 (0) 870 240 1239
www.petsastherapy.org

RUGMARK UK
Address as for Anti-Slavery International
Tel: +44 (0) 20 7737 2675
www.rugmark.org

USEFUL ADDRESSES

Soil Association
Bristol House,
40-56 Victoria Street
Bristol BS1 6BY, UK
Tel: +44 (0) 117 914 2444
www.soilassociation.org

Viva! Vegetarians' International Voice for Animals
8 York Court, Wilder street
Bristol BS2 8QH, UK
Tel: +44 (0) 117 944 1000
www.viva.org.uk
www.vivausa.org

Women's Environmental Network
PO Box 30626
London E1 1TZ, UK
Tel:+44 (0) 20 7481 9004
www.wen.org.uk

USA

Co-op America
1612 K Street NW
Suite 600
Washington DC 20006
Tel: (800) 854 7336
www.coopamerica.org

Free the Slaves
1012 14th Street NW
Suite 600
Washington DC 2005
Tel: 202 638 1865
www.freetheslaves.net

Humane society of the United States (Animal Compassion Foundation)
2100 L Street NW
Washington DC 20037
Tel: 202 452 1100
www.hsus.org
www.animalcompassionfoundation.org

National Organic Program
Dept. of Agriculture
USDA-AMS-TMP-NOP
Room 4008 South Building
1400 Independence Avenue SW
Washington DC
20250-0020
Tel: 202 720 3252
www.ams.usda.gov/NOP

Pesticide Action Network North America (PANNA)
49 Powell Street
Suite 500
San Francisco
CA 94102
Tel: 415 981 1771
www.panna.org

People for the Ethical Treatment of Animals (PETA)
501 Front Street
Norfolk VA 77510
Tel: 757-627-PETA (7382)
Info@peta.org

RUGMARK Foundation
20001 3 Street NW
Suite 430
Washington DC 20009USA
Tel 202 234 9050
www.rugmark.org

Social Investment Forum
1612 K Street NW
Suite 650
Washington DC 20006
Tel: 202 872 5319
www.socialinvest.org

Transfair USA
1611 Telegraph Avenue
Suite 900
Oakland CA 94612
info@transfairusa.org
www.transfairusa.org

INDEX

acoustic insulation 78
ActionAid 115-116
addiction 46
Aggression 74, 100, 102
aid 112, 113
AIDS 66, 134
air 79, 84, 122
air filters 15
Air fresheners 19, 74
alchemy 2, 142
allopathic 39
Alpha Hydroxy Acids 23
Alzheimer's 22, 24, 27, 134
anger 51, 60, 102
animal testing 133-136
animal welfare 34, 131-132
animals 34, 75, 84, 99, 130-131, 134-137, 142
anti-oxidant vitamins 24, 28
Anti-slavery International 114
anti-social behaviour 101
antibiotics 24, 132
anxiety 84
appliances 12, 14-15, 35-36, 77, 107, 127
asthma 3
astronomy 153
atmosphere 61, 69, 104, 122, 124-125
attention 99-100
attention deficit disorders 27
aura 56
autumn 148
avian flu 131

Babbit, Edwin 55
baby 60, 70, 145
backache 24, 33, 35
balance 1, 29, 60-62, 92, 123, 145-146
bathroom 20, 64, 73, 83
beauty 21, 24
bed 36
bedroom 20, 52, 64, 72-73, 89
behaviour 100-101 108, 120, 145, 160-161
Bell, J.S. 160
Beltane 147
bio-electrical energy 75
bio-piracy 115
biophysics 66

birds 84, 139, 141-143
Birren, Faber 55
bloating 33
blood pressure 58
Boirac 56
brain 32, 50, 52, 54, 63-64, 70-71, 73, 77
Breathing 87
Brigantia 151
British Medical Journal, The 28
British Union for the Abolition of
    Vivisection 136
Brown, Lancelot 'Capability' 121
BSE 27
business 101, 111
butter 29
butterflies 140

cancer 3, 21-22, 24, 27, 41, 46, 55, 85, 93, 134,
    146, 150
Candlemas 152
candles 81-82
capitalism 93
car 125
carbon dioxide 123, 124
carbon monoxide 14
carpet industry 116, 118
cash-crop 112, 115, 121
Celts 146-151
central nervous system 44
chairs 37-38
chakras 56-57
Chamomile 76
Chartres 48
chemicals 6, 13-14, 16, 24, 28, 31, 81, 121, 133,
    138
Children 12, 14, 18, 21, 60, 70, 75-76, 99-101,
    104-106, 109, 116, 118, 136
chimes 78, 86, 87
chimneys 13-14, 53, 81, 85
chocolate 113, 118
Christ 56
Christian 93, 138, 149, 152-153
Christmas 141, 149
cigarette smoke 15
circadian rhythm 65, 144
clatter 77-78

cleaning *16-20, 81*
cleaning agents *74*
Climate Change *125*
clutter *37, 50-52, 71, 90*
Co-operative Bank *111, 119*
coffee *113, 115, 118*
Colour *54-56, 58-59, 64, 73, 80, 82-83, 88, 105,*
   154,
comfort *35, 48, 50, 52, 99*
Committee of Publication Ethics *28*
Communism *93*
community *99, 103, 106, 109-110*
Companion planting *139*
Compassion In World Farming *132*
compost *8, 53*
computers *5, 8, 37, 64, 69*
connection *3, 47, 63, 91, 95, 102, 138, 142, 162*
conscience *99*
consciousness *98*
constipation *24, 33*
consumers *7, 30-31, 113, 118, 132*
contact dermatitis *21*
control *77-78, 107*
convenience *7, 32, 133*
Cork, Dr Michael *23*
Council, Forest Stewardship *7*
creativity *87, 89*
cruelty free products *136*
crystal *56, 80, 82*
Curtains *6, 67, 85*

D.I.Y *1, 77*
DDT *27*
de-humidifiers *15*
De-scaling *19*
death *61, 92, 151*
decision-making *106*
decoration *49, 88, 150*
depression *12, 65*
design *35, 48, 53-54, 72*
detergents *17*
detoxification *147*
diabetes *3, 134*
diarrhoea *33*
Dimmer switches *69*
Dining rooms *63, 72, 104*
disease *39, 93, 131, 133*
dishwasher *36*

double-glazing *78*
Drains *19*
drug industry *39*
Druids *146*
dusting *19*

Earth *79-80, 120-122 148, 150, 152-154*
Easter *152*
eating *32-34, 39*
eczema *23*
Einstein, Albert *157*
electricity *83, 124*
electromagnetism *15, 54-55, 156*
elements *79, 81-82, 84*
Emoto, Masaru Dr. *33, 130*
Energy; colour *54, 55, 88*
Energy; cosmic *154*
Energy; efficiency *7, 14, 18, 68, 81, 124*
Energy; field *55, 56*
Energy; light *54, 55, 65, 66*
Energy; seasonal *144-152*
environment *5-9, 120-129*
ergonomic assessment *35, 72*
essential fatty acids *29*
Essential oils *18-20, 74-76*
ethical credentials *7*
ethical investment *119*
Euclid *48*
Exercise *25, 49, 125, 158*
exploitation *102, 114-117, 119-122*
eye-strain *64, 69*

fabric *14, 62, 85, 73*
fabric softener *17*
Face pack *25*
Facial scrub *25*
fair-trade *115*
Fairtrade Foundation *117-118*
faith *3, 91, 93, 158-159*
family *32, 49, 60, 62, 99-106, 149, 159*
farming *27, 130*
fatigue *24, 35, 65*
Fawkes, Guy *149*
fear *1, 34, 45-46, 51, 72, 74, 92, 94, 158*
feng shui *61, 91, 145*
fertility *27, 147, 152*
fertilizers *27, 92, 121*
festivals *81, 109, 146, 148-152*

fibreboard *13*
filtering system *52, 54, 77, 107*
fire *79, 81-82, 149*
fireplace *53, 81*
fish-reserves *122*
fits *12*
flooring *13-14, 19, 72-73, 77*
flowers *61, 74, 88*
fluoride *21-22*
food *27-33, 63, 66, 130*
forest *121-122*
Forest Stewardship Council *127*
formaldehyde *12-13*
fossil fuels *122*
fridge/freezers *36*
front door *87*
furnishings *49-50, 73, 77*
furniture *6, 15, 35, 52, 72, 105,*

garages *14*
garden waste *108, 127*
gardens *49, 108, 138-142*
garlic *140-141*
gastric pain *16*
gemstones *55*
gender *73*
genetic damage *22*
Geranium *75, 141*
global temperatures *123*
globalization *111*
Glycerin *22*
God *98, 145*
Golden Section *48*
Grace *34*
grants *129*
Greenpeace Environmental Trust *31*

Hair rinse *26*
Hairspray *26*
Hand and body moisturizer *26*
happiness *3-4, 44, 47, 51, 89, 99, 130, 137, 159*
hardwoods *121*
harmony *53, 60, 95, 102, 144, 157, 159*
headaches *24, 35, 39*
healing *33-34, 40-41, 148, 154, 158-159*
health *2, 4, 24, 34, 39, 41, 47, 66, 130, 133, 145, 157-159*
heart *53, 56-57, 82*

heart attack *137*
Heart disease *3, 29, 46, 85, 146*
heating *81, 124*
helio-therapy *65*
herbs *140*
Hinduism *153*
HIV *134*
hobbies *49*
holistic health *2, 39, 41, 44, 46, 93-94, 127, 140, 162*
honesty *94, 100, 162*
hormonal system *44, 55, 93*
hormones *23-24, 27, 39, 46, 65, 144*
household products *16, 130, 135*
housework *105*
human rights *114, 116, 119*
Humphrys, John *27*
hydrogenated fats *29*
hygiene *16*
hypocrisy *100*

imagery *79, 84*
Imbolc *151*
immune systems *15-17, 47, 65, 75, 131, 148*
inclusion *101, 104-105*
insects *19, 84, 142*
insomnia *15, 39*
inspiration *81, 87, 89-90*
insulation *77-78, 107*
intelligence *30, 160-161*
intensive farming *27, 92, 122, 130, 132*
intention *158-159, 162*
interaction *2, 49, 53, 56*
Intergovernmental Panel *125*
International Monetary Fund *102, 112*
internet *7*
intuition *48, 99*
investment *1, 104, 106, 108, 158*
ionizers *15*
irritability *12, 39*
irritable bowel *39*
Islamic *93*

joint pain *15, 24*

kidney damage *22*
kindness *33, 137, 162*
Kirlian, Semyon *56*

kitchen *18, 35, 63, 72, 105*
Kuhn, Thomas *155, 161*

Lammas *148*
Lancet, The *28*
landfill *5*
laundry *20*
laundry detergent *17*
Lavender *18, 63, 76*
Le Corbusier *48*
Lemon *18, 75*
Lemon balm *140*
lethargy *12, 15, 39, 65*
Liebeault *56*
light *54, 65-67, 162*
lighting *67-69*
Lime *13, 18*
Lime-scale *20*
love *32, 74, 89, 94, 100, 158*
Low-level grills *36*
Lughnassadh *148*
lymphatic system *39*

magic *82, 147, 152*
margarine *29*
Marine Stewardship Council *127*
marriage *145, 147*
massage *25*
Material Safety Data Sheet *16, 22-23*
materialism *2*
mattress *36*
May Day *147*
McNicholas, Dr June *136*
mealtimes *105*
meat *34, 121, 130, 132*
meditation *25, 34, 60, 89, 158*
memorabilia *51*
memory problems *22, 24*
meningitis *131*
Meteorological Office *122*
methane *6, 122*
mice *19*
mind/body connection *40, 44-45*
minerals *24, 28-29, 148*
Mintel *32*
mobile phones *6, 8*
Moon *20, 82, 144, 151-154*
moral *99, 101, 103*

morphic fields *161*
Moth repellent *20*
mould *20*
Muslims *138*

nappies *7*
natural gypsum *13*
nature *72, 91, 94, 138, 142, 146-147*
nausea *12, 16*
negotiation *105*
neighbours *77-78, 107-109*
neo-natal jaundice *68*
nettles *140*
neurological impairment *16, 22*
New Year *148*
Newton, Isaac *156*
nocebo *40-41*
noise *72, 77-78, 107*
non-toxic fibreboards *13*
non-toxic paints *13, 80*
nutrition *28-29, 33, 55, 80, 148, 158*

obesity *3, 46, 85*
Oestra *152*
office *37*
olfactory nerves *73*
optic nerve *54*
organic *30-31, 34, 127, 132*
organic farming *118*
organic food *31, 81, 118*
organochlorine *27*
organophosphates *27*
orientation *66, 154*
osteoporosis *85*
Oxfam *112*

pack behaviour *99-100*
packaging *8, 126*
pain *34, 39, 51, 92, 135*
painkillers *39*
paint *8, 12-13, 62, 80, 85, 127*
panaceas *91*
parasites *24*
parasympathetic nervous system *46*
parasympathetic reaction *45*
parents *60, 100-101, 104-106*
Parkinson's *27, 134*
parlour games *151*

Parsley *140*
perfume *74*
peripheral nervous system (PNS) *44*
personal care *21, 135*
pessimism *46*
Pesticide Action Network *138*
pesticides *14, 27, 31, 138-139*
pets *21, 136*
Pets As Therapy *136*
pheromones *73*
photodynamic therapy *66*
photons *66*
photosynthesis *65*
physics *156*
physiological reactions *45*
Pine *18*
pineal *65*
pituitary *65*
placebos *40-41 91*
plants *15, 74, 139-140*
plaster *12*
Plato *48*
play *104*
Pliny *55*
pneumonia *131*
polish *19*
pollution *6, 8, 28, 84, 126*
Poly-Vinyl Chloride *88*
poor concentration *12*
Popp, Fritz-Albert *66, 130*
possessions *50-51, 86*
power *1, 41, 94, 98, 128, 153, 159, 162*
prayer *34*
presents *151*
processed foods *32*
Propylene glycol *23*
psoriasis *68*
psychological breakdown *46*

quantum theory *157*
Querencia *79*

Ransom, Steve *41*
re-birth *93, 142, 150-152*
recycling *6, 8, 51*
refrigerators *18*
relationship *49, 83, 100, 107, 120, 130*
relaxation *1, 24, 87, 89*

religion *44, 98*
renewable resources *123-124*
research *27-28, 133, 155, 159*
research laboratories *92, 130*
research misconduct *28*
resonance *76, 111, 161*
respect *89, 94, 162*
respiratory infections *12, 16*
responsibility *46, 101-102, 111, 123-124, 129,
    159, 161-162*
rituals *32, 145, 150-151*
room deodorizers *74*
Rosemary *141*
RUGMARK' *118*
Rust *20*

Sacred Geometry *48-49*
safe houses *109*
Sage *141*
salmonella *131*
Samhain *148-149*
Scent *73-76*
scientists *28, 130, 155*
screening *78*
sea *84, 122*
Seasonal Affective Disorder (SAD Syn-
    drome) *65, 144*
seasons *144-152*
self-respect *106*
self-responsibility *46, 124*
senses *70-78*
Sheldrake, Rupert *160*
Shinto *138*
Showers *126*
sick building syndrome *12*
Sinks *18*
sitting room *63*
slavery *113-114*
Sleep *24, 36*
slugs *141*
Smell *70-71, 73-74*
snails *141*
society *3, 92, 95, 99-100, 145, 155-156, 160*
sociopathic *101*
sodium laureth sulphate *22*
Sodium Lauryl Sulphate *22*
soft furnishings *77*
soil *28, 92, 122*

Soil Association *132*
solstice *150*
solvents *17*
Soul *83*
Sound *76-77*
spirit *98, 145-146, 152, 159, 162*
sports teams *109*
spring *145, 147, 151-152*
spring cleaning *39, 147*
stainless steel *50, 72*
staircases *72, 108*
stomach problems *22*
stone *72, 80*
Stonehenge *153*
storage *36*
stress *3, 33, 35, 45-47, 68, 107, 131*
stress response *1*
stroke *137*
Structural Adjustment Programmes *112*
summer *52, 145, 147-148*
Sun *20, 150, 152-154, 147-148*
sunlight *62, 65-66, 68, 85*
Supermarkets *8, 31, 131-132*
Superstring *76*
sustainability *92, 103, 118, 122, 144*
sutras *76*
sympathetic nervous system *45-46*
sympathetic reaction *45*
synthetic drugs *39-40*

tables *63, 105*
talismans *53*
Tea tree *18, 76*
television *5, 69, 82, 105*
textiles *6, 12, 14, 62, 73, 113, 116, 127*
textures *72-73, 80*
Thames Water Utilities *125*
Thyme *141*
toilet cleaners *17*
toothpaste *21*
touch *71*
toxins *5, 12-13, 15, 23-24, 27-28*
trade *111-115, 117*
trade barriers *113*
Trade Related Aspects of Intellectual
    Property Rights *116*
truth *82, 91, 94, 155*
tuberculosis *65*

UN Food and Agriculture Organization
    122
Union Carbide *123*
US Environmental Protection Agency
    (EPA) *12*

vCJD *27*
Veda *76*
ventilation *13-14, 85*
vibrancy *52*
vibrations *33-34, 55, 71, 76, 130, 161*
violence *63*
vitamins *28-29, 55, 65*
Viva! *131*
vivisection *134-135*
volatile organic compounds *13*

War, Second World *27*
waste *6, 126, 139*
water *24, 33, 78-79, 82-84, 125-126, 141*
water crystals *33, 130*
Water-Wise *126*
Watson, Lyall *160*
weather *128*
wind ornaments *78, 85*
Window boxes *138, 140, 142*
Windows *19, 67, 78, 85*
winter *52, 65, 139, 141, 145, 150-151*
Women's Environmental Network *7*
wood *7, 14, 50, 72, 80, 88, 142*
work *32, 64, 89, 105, 144*
work surfaces *35-36, 68*
Workstations *37*
worktops *18*
World Bank *102, 112*
World Development Movement *113*
World Health Organization *162*
World Trade Organization *102, 112, 116*
World Wildlife Fund *128*

yoga *25*
Youth *101, 110*
Yule Log *150*